Bravehearts

Men's Guide to Heart Health and Stroke Prevention

By
Well-Being Publishing

To You,

Thank you!

Contents

Introduction 1

Chapter 1: Understanding Heart Health 4
    The Anatomy of the Heart... 4
    How the Heart Works 7
    Risk Factors for Heart Disease 11

Chapter 2: Recognizing the Enemy: An Overview of Heart Disease 14
    Types of Heart Diseases... 14
    Statistics and Why Men Are at Risk............................ 17
    The Impact of Age, Genetics, and Ethnicity 17

Chapter 3: The Warning Signs and Symptoms of Heart Disease 22
    Recognizing a Heart Attack 22
    Symptoms of Stroke.. 25
    When to Seek Emergency Care 28

Chapter 4: The Stroke Connection................................... 31
    Understanding Stroke... 31
    Prevention and Recovery Strategies............................ 34
    The Role of Rehabilitation in Stroke Recovery 35

Chapter 5: Lifestyle Choices for Heart Health 39
    Quitting Smoking 39
    Managing Stress 42
    The Importance of Sleep 45

Chapter 6: Nutrition for a Healthy Heart 48
    Heart-Healthy Diet Basics.. 48

Foods to Eat and Avoid 51

The Role of Supplements in Heart Health 52

Chapter 7: Exercise Your Way to a Stronger Heart 55

Benefits of Regular Exercise 55

Creating a Personalized Exercise Plan 58

Staying Motivated for Long-Term Success 59

Chapter 8: Tackling Obesity and Weight Management..... 63

The Link Between Weight and Heart Health 63

Strategies for Losing Weight Safely 66

Tracking Progress and Setting Realistic Goals 67

Chapter 9: Managing Blood Pressure and Cholesterol..... 71

Understanding Blood Pressure Numbers 72

Strategies for Managing High Cholesterol 74

The Importance of Regular Health Screenings.................. 75

Chapter 10: Understanding and Managing Diabetes 79

Diabetes and Heart Disease Connection 79

Lifestyle Management for Diabetics 82

Monitoring and Medication Compliance 83

Chapter 11: Alcohol, Drugs, and Heart Health 86

The Effects of Alcohol on the Heart.................................... 86

The Dangers of Recreational Drug Use............................... 89

Seeking Help for Substance Abuse 90

Chapter 12: Mental Health and Its Impact on Heart Health 94

The Connection Between Mental Health and Heart Disease 94

Stress Management Techniques... 97

Coping with Heart Disease: Psychological Aspects 98

Chapter 13: Empowering Your Heart-Healthy Journey.................. 101

Appendix A: Heart-Healthy Recipes 104

Hearty Oatmeal with Berries and Nuts.............................. 104

Grilled Salmon with Steamed Broccoli 105

Quinoa and Black Bean Salad 105

Vegetable Stir-Fry Over Brown Rice 105

Appendix B: Recommended Exercise Routines 107

Getting Started 107

Low-Intensity Exercises 107

Moderate-Intensity Exercises 108

Strength Training 108

Flexibility and Balance 108

Examples of Strength Training Exercises 109

Consistency is Key 109

Appendix C: Resources for Heart Health and Support Groups 110

National and International Organizations 110

Support Networks and Groups 110

Online Resources and Tools 111

Apps and Tech for Heart Health 111

Educational Books and Materials 112

Counseling and Therapy 112

In Conclusion 112

Introduction

Welcome to a journey that is both critical and empowering, a journey that speaks to the very rhythm of life—your heart health. This text is dedicated to exploring the intricacies of the heart, the majesty of its functions, and the caution one must take to protect this vital organ. As we delve into the pages that lie ahead, remember that your heart is not only a biological wonder but also a symbol of your connection to others and to life itself.

You're not alone in this journey. Whether you are a man with heart disease, a health-conscious individual, a caregiver, or a healthcare professional, these pages are crafted to provide insights and guidance tailored to improve heart health. But beyond facts and advice, this book aims to kindle a flame of motivation within, inspiring you to take charge and make enduring changes for a healthier heart.

Understanding how your heart works is the bedrock of preventative health. With knowledge comes power—the power to recognize risk factors and the power to make informed decisions that can steer you clear of the perils of heart disease. This book isn't simply about absorbing information; it's about translating that information into actions that fit seamlessly into your life.

The data surrounding heart disease can be startling. Being equipped with the reality of the risks and understanding why certain groups, particularly men, are at a higher risk can help galvanize change. But it's the synthesis of this knowledge with personalized insight that truly fosters transformation. Age, genetics, and ethnicity all play a role in heart health, but none are determinants of destiny.

Recognizing the warning signs and symptoms of heart disease is your first line of defense. It's paramount to understand what a heart attack feels like, how to spot the onset of a stroke, and when it's time to seek emergency care. Awareness can mean the difference between life and death, and immediate action can save precious heart muscle and brain function.

Moreover, heart health and stroke prevention are intrinsically linked. This book will guide you through understanding the connection, as well as strategies for prevention and recovery. With dedication and persistence, it's possible to navigate the road to recovery and reclaim a fulfilling life post-stroke.

Long-term heart health is influenced by the lifestyle decisions that we make each day. Simple choices have complex outcomes, from opting to quit smoking to effectively managing stress. Moreover, the importance of sleep cannot be understated—it's during those restful hours that your heart gets a chance to recuperate and prepare for the challenges of the following day.

The foods we eat are the building blocks of our bodily health. Nutrition is a cornerstone of a heart-healthy lifestyle. Through these chapters, you will learn about diet fundamentals, which foods to embrace, and which to avoid. The aim is to arm you with the knowledge to make meal choices that support a robust, beating heart.

Exercise isn't just about losing weight; it's about strengthening the most important muscle you have. Regular physical activity keeps the heart resilient and responsive. You will be equipped to craft an exercise plan that resonates with you—one that not only suits your current fitness level but also evolves with your progress and maintains your long-term health.

Obesity has been unequivocally linked to heart health troubles. Within these pages, you will find strategies not just to lose weight, but to manage it effectively and sustainably. You'll learn to set achievable goals and track your journey towards a weight that keeps your heart functioning at its best.

High blood pressure and cholesterol are silent adversaries in the quest for a healthy heart. Understanding these numbers and knowing how to manage them can protect you from heart disease's stealthy advance. Together with regular health screenings, you'll formulate a fortified defense against the unforeseen.

Diabetes presents a unique challenge to heart health, touching every aspect of your journey towards wellness. Managing diabetes requires vigilance, a proactive attitude towards lifestyle management, and compliance with necessary medications. Untangling the knot between heart disease and diabetes is vital to protecting your heart's future.

Substances such as alcohol and recreational drugs have a deleterious effect on your heart. This book confronts these dangers head-on, offering strategies to reduce intake and providing a path towards seeking help if substance abuse has taken hold. In protecting your heart, you're also guarding the essence of your vitality and life's potential.

Your mental health is as instrumental to your heart's wellbeing as any medication or lifestyle change. The intricate connection between your mental state and heart disease cannot be overlooked. Stress management and adapting to life with heart disease are not just about coping; they are about thriving in the face of adversity.

In conclusion, the blueprint for a heart-healthy life is within these pages. With every day that passes, the choices you make carve deeper habits and a reverence for the life that beats in your chest. It's time to empower your heart-healthy journey, so let's begin with a single, hopeful beat—a step towards a future of wellness and vitality.

Chapter 1:
Understanding Heart Health

Embarking on the journey towards heart health, it's crucial to grasp the fundamentals; the cornerstone being an understanding of the heart itself. Imagine your heart as the diligent engine in the center of your intricate cardiovascular system, tirelessly pumping life-sustaining blood through a maze of vessels. Here, we'll delve into the anatomy of this remarkable organ, highlighting its chambers, valves, and the symphony of electrical impulses that maintain a steady rhythm. You'll learn how these components work in unison to fuel every cell in your body. Understanding the elements at play behind every beat lays the groundwork for recognizing how lifestyle choices impact the intricate workings of your heart. Knowledge about risk factors is your first line of defense – acting not as a harbinger of limitations, but as a beacon guiding you towards a life nurtured by informed, heart-conscious decisions. Remember, the power to invigorate your heart health rests in your hands; knowing the essence of your heart's function is the initial stride on a transformative path toward vigor and longevity.

The Anatomy of the Heart

Embarking on a journey to improve heart health begins with a foundational understanding of the heart's anatomy. The heart, a marvel of biological engineering, is the cornerstone of the cardiovascular system. Each beat sustains life, sending blood coursing through veins and arteries to nourish every cell in the body. Without it functioning properly, all systems falter. So, what makes the heart an incredible powerhouse at the center of our circulatory system?

The heart is essentially a muscular pump divided into four chambers: the upper chambers are called atria and the lower chambers are known as ventricles. The right atrium receives deoxygenated blood from the body and pumps it into the right ventricle, which in turn, sends it to the lungs to be oxygenated. The left atrium receives this oxygen-rich blood from the lungs and transfers it to the left ventricle, where it is then pumped out to the rest of the body.

Valves within these chambers ensure blood flows in a single direction: the tricuspid valve between the right atrium and ventricle, the pulmonary valve leading to the lungs, the mitral valve between the left atrium and ventricle, and the aortic valve leading to the body. These valves open and close with the heart's rhythm, preventing backflow and keeping blood moving efficiently on its life-sustaining path.

Surrounding the heart is a protective sac called the pericardium. This double-layered membrane cushions the heart and contains a small amount of fluid to reduce friction between the heart and surrounding tissues as the heart beats.

The heart wall itself is made up of three layers: the endocardium (inner layer), the myocardium (middle and thickest layer consisting of heart muscle), and the epicardium (outer layer). The myocardium is responsible for the contraction of the heart, making it the workhorse that drives blood through your body.

The heart's own blood supply is fascinatingly self-supporting—coronary arteries run along the heart's surface, providing it with the oxygen-rich blood it needs to function. These vessels play a critical role, as any blockage can lead to serious health consequences, such as a heart attack.

Electrical impulses within the heart's conduction system initiate each heartbeat. Starting in the sinoatrial (SA) node, located in the right atrium, electrical signals then spread through the atria, causing them to contract and push blood into the ventricles. The impulse then reaches the atrioventricular (AV) node, pausing briefly to allow the ventricles to fill before it causes them to contract and propel blood onward.

Anatomy is destiny, particularly when it comes to the heart. Individual variation in heart structure can influence both function and health. For instance, some people are born with congenital heart defects, which can affect how their heart handles blood flow and can have a significant impact on overall health.

Understanding the heart's anatomy empowers us not only with knowledge but also with intentional respect for this vital organ. The heart is not only a symbol of life but also an embodiment of resilience, tirelessly adapting to the demands we place upon it. Its well-coordinated structure and function remind us that the health we take for granted hinges on a delicate balance.

Our lifestyle choices can significantly influence heart function. Choices around diet, exercise, and stress management directly impact the cardiovascular system's health and efficiency. Positive changes in these areas lead to stronger heart muscles, improved circulation, and a reduced risk of heart-related issues.

As we learn about the heart's anatomy, we can visualize how every action—from the food we consume to the level of physical activity we engage in—has an immediate impact on our heart's health. We create a ripple effect that can enhance or harm our well-being based on our daily decisions.

Consider the heart as the body's CEO, with a never-ending work ethic. Even at rest, it works diligently, beating approximately 100,000 times a day, moving an estimated 2,000 gallons of blood daily. When we're active, these numbers increase exponentially. Thus, maintaining the health of this executive organ is crucial to maintain the efficient operation of our body's systems.

Exploring the greater depths of heart anatomy and physiology reveals a road map to understanding what our heart needs for optimal performance. While the heart is strong, it is also vulnerable to damage, which can be cumulative and irreversible. Prevention, therefore, becomes a paramount strategy in maintaining heart health and preventing disease—a proactive approach that will be further explored in this book.

Finally, appreciation for the heart's anatomy is completed with an acknowledgment of its symbolic strength. Across cultures and ages, the heart has been recognized for its representation of love, courage, and endurance—qualities necessary not just for health, but for the fullness of human experience.

As we travel through each page, let this be a heartfelt reminder: take care of your heart, and it will take care of you. Every heartbeat is a miracle—let's strive to protect and strengthen this vital pulse with the wisdom and tools we have. Your journey towards heart health is one of the most significant investments you'll ever make; as you support your heart, you support every aspect of your life.

How the Heart Works

The heart, an engineering marvel inside the human body, is nothing short of extraordinary in its form and function. The essence of its purpose can be summarized simply: the heart pumps blood throughout the body, delivering oxygen and nutrients to tissues and removing wastes. Yet, this core function underpins our very existence. Understanding how your heart works is the first step towards taking command of your heart health.

Let's envision the heart as a dedicated power house, divided into four chambers: the two upper chambers, the atria, and the two lower chambers, the ventricles. These chambers work in a harmonious symphony to keep blood circulating in a methodical pattern. As blood returns from the body, depleted of oxygen, it enters the right atrium. From there, it flows into the right ventricle, which propels it into the lungs to be replenished with life-sustaining oxygen.

Once the blood has traversed the lung's alveoli and embraced fresh oxygen, it journeys back to the heart, but this time to the left atrium. The saga continues as blood descends into the mighty left ventricle, the chamber with the herculean task of launching it throughout the vast network of arteries, delivering that precious oxygen to every corner of your body.

The orchestration between these chambers is regulated by a system of valves - tricuspid, pulmonary, mitral, and aortic - each acting like a gate that ensures blood flows in the right direction, preventing any backflow. Timing is crucial here. Valves open to permit blood flow from one chamber to another or into an artery and then close tightly to stop blood from flowing backward.

This rhythmic dance is set in motion by an electrical impulse, initially generated in a cluster of cells known as the sinoatrial node, or the heart's natural pacemaker. This electrical signal spreads through the atria, signaling them to contract and push blood into the ventricles. Then, it travels to the atrioventricular node, and after a brief pause, prompts the ventricles to contract. This sequence of contraction, coordinated by these electrical pulses, results in the heartbeat you can feel at your wrist or chest - the reassuring thump-thump that accompanies you every moment of your life.

Doesn't it instill a sense of wonder to think that the heart's rhythm is maintained 24/7 by this finely tuned electrical system? In the average lifetime, this amounts to an astonishing three billion beats! But to sustain such a high level of performance, the heart itself needs a relentless supply of blood. Enter the coronary arteries, the vessels tasked with feeding the heart muscle.

Just as roads can become blocked, so too can these essential arteries, and that's where risk factors for heart disease come into play. Lifestyle, diet, and genetics all contribute to the integrity of these arteries. Keeping them clear and functioning is a vital aspect of heart health, because any blockage can disrupt the flow of oxygen to the heart, potentially leading to a heart attack - something we must be vigilant to avoid.

Aside from blood movement and electrical impulses, the heart's work involves maintaining an exquisite balance with other body systems. It dynamically adjusts to the demands of your daily activities, whether you're asleep or running a marathon. When you're exercising, for example, your heart rate increases to supply more oxygen rapidly to your muscles. Resting sees the heart pace slowing down, conserving energy and allowing the body to recover.

Blood pressure is a term you're undoubtedly familiar with, and it plays a significant role in how the heart operates. When the heart beats, it creates pressure that pushes blood through a network of tube-shaped vessels, including arteries, veins, and capillaries. This pressure is necessary for the blood to reach the body's farthest reaches. However, elevated blood pressure over time can stress the heart and contribute to plaque buildup, offering us yet another reason to maintain a healthy lifestyle that promotes optimal circulatory function.

Understanding that heart health isn't isolated, but intertwined with other aspects of your wellness, is foundational. For instance, your kidneys help regulate blood pressure, which in turn affects the workload on your heart. Inflammation in the body can influence the health of your arteries and thus affect heart function. Seeing the body as an interconnected web, with the heart at its center, enables a more holistic approach to wellness.

Your heart's endurance is nothing short of phenomenal, yet it requires care, much like a prized possession. Protecting your heart means being conscious of what goes into your body, the activities you engage in, and the environment around you. Nurturing your heart with wholesome foods, regular physical activity, and stress management techniques isn't just an act of maintenance—it's a profound expression of respect for the vital organ that keeps you alive.

Let's not overlook the impact of the mind on heart health. Negative emotions like stress, anger, and anxiety can accelerate the heart rate and raise blood pressure, exacerbating the wear on your heart. Cultivating a positive mindset and emotional resilience can therefore be seen as a boon to your cardiovascular system.

As we conclude this exploration of how the heart works, embrace the understanding that your heart is more than just a biological wonder; it's the very engine of life. With every beat, it testifies to your existence, your experiences, your emotions. In caring for your heart, you're not simply looking after an organ; you're honoring your own life story and all the vibrance it contains.

Now that you're equipped with knowledge of how your heart works, let that empower and motivate you to make choices that reflect the awe and respect this remarkable organ deserves. Your heart's health is in your hands; tender it with the care that befits the guardian of your vitality.

Every heart deserves a chance to keep beating strongly and healthily. Yours is no exception. Use this newfound understanding as a foundation to build upon, as we move forward into the next chapters discussing risk factors and preventative measures for heart health. Remember, knowledge is power, and with great power comes great responsibility - the responsibility to take action and advocate for the health of your heart.

Risk Factors for Heart Disease

Grasping the intricacies of heart health is incomplete without a deep understanding of the risk factors for heart disease. These are the conditions and lifestyles that set the stage for potential cardiac challenges. Some you're born with, while others creep in through choices and circumstances. They're critical to identify and, where possible, mitigate. Let's dive into these factors and discuss practical steps for minimizing their impact.

The very blueprint of who we are, our genetics, is a risk factor that we have little control over. If heart disease runs in your family, you might be predisposed to conditions that put your heart at risk. Even though we can't alter our genetics, knowing this risk can empower you to take more rigorous preventative actions in other areas.

Age is another factor beyond our immediate control. Simply put, the older you get, the higher your risk of heart disease. One cannot stop the march of time, but one can age with grace and strength by adopting heart-conscious lifestyle adjustments.

Elevated blood pressure, or hypertension, is a stealthy adversary that often slips by unnoticed. It exerts undue strain on your arteries and heart, which can lead to damage over time. Monitoring your blood pressure and managing it through diet, exercise, and medication when necessary is essential.

Cholesterol levels in your blood are like a double-edged sword. While some cholesterol is necessary for your body's workings, excess levels, especially of 'bad' LDL cholesterol, can lead to artery-clogging plaque. Keeping cholesterol in check is basic heart defense.

Diabetes is a significant risk factor that doubles the likelihood of heart disease. High blood sugar can damage arteries and set the groundwork for atherosclerosis. Managing diabetes and maintaining healthy blood sugar levels is tantamount to protecting your heart.

Smoking — an absolute nemesis to your heart. It damages your blood vessels, reduces oxygen in your blood, and raises blood pressure — a cocktail of risks. If you've taken up the habit, quitting is perhaps one of the best things you can do for your heart.

Obesity carries with it a heavy burden of risk. Excess weight, especially around the midsection, is linked to high blood pressure, diabetes, and lipid problems, all of which stress the heart. Shedding even a moderate amount of weight can have significant health returns.

Don't overlook physical inactivity — it's often termed the 'new smoking' due to its profound link to heart disease. Regular physical activity is key, so make it a daily goal to stay moving and push back against heart risks.

It's not just substances such as tobacco that wield a heavy sword; excessive alcohol consumption can also hike up blood pressure, cause heart muscle damage, and contribute to other heart-related issues. Moderation is paramount.

While we often think of diet as related to weight, it also stands alone as a risk factor. A diet high in saturated fat, trans fat, salt, and sugar can propel you towards heart disease, whereas a heart-healthy diet can be your fortress.

Stress is not just felt mentally; it's physically embodied and can impact your heart. Chronic stress has been linked with hypertension and other heart risks. Managing stress is not a luxury; it's a necessary element of heart disease prevention.

We come to understand that not all risk factors are penned in black and white — some are interwoven with social determinants of health, such as socio-economic status, access to healthcare, and educational inequalities. Addressing these broader social issues can be a daunting task, but it is essential as a community health initiative.

Your sleep habits also hold a piece of the heart health puzzle. Poor sleep has been linked to higher risks of heart disease. Restorative sleep can do wonders for regulating blood pressure and overall heart health.

Lastly, illicit drug use poses serious risks to cardiovascular health. Drugs like cocaine can cause arrhythmias and heart attacks, and anabolic steroids can increase cholesterol levels. Steering clear of these substances protects your heart's well-being.

Recognizing and acknowledging these risk factors is your first step toward a healthier heart. With every tweak in your lifestyle choices, you strengthen your heart against the wave of potential ailments. It's a steady journey toward wellness, and every choice you make builds a future where your heart can thrive. Take control, not just for yourself, but for those who share your journey. Your heart's health is your life's rhythm, keep it strong, keep it steady, and cherish it with every beat.

Chapter 2:
Recognizing the Enemy:
An Overview of Heart Disease

Emerging from the foundational insights of heart anatomy and function, the journey continues with a crucial chapter that confronts the formidable adversary—heart disease. Grasping the full scope of this enemy is the first step toward empowerment. This chapter endeavors to not only inform but also to ignite a sense of urgency and determination. While heart disease takes on many forms, from the silent progression of atherosclerosis to the sudden onset of myocardial infarction, the underlying feature is its stealthy prowess in undermining heart health. It's an affliction that sees no bias, touching lives across every social stratum and geography. Throughout this section, we'll examine the extent of its reach, unwrap the stark statistics, and unveil why men, in particular, find themselves in the crosshairs of this relentless condition. By recognizing heart disease for what it truly is—a beatable foe when faced with knowledge, resolve, and actionable health strategies—we can begin to dismantle the barriers to a robust heart and reclaim the vitality we deserve.

Types of Heart Diseases

As we advance in our understanding of heart health, it's important to focus on the multifaceted enemy we're up against. Heart disease is not a singular condition but rather a collection of disorders affecting the heart and blood vessels. Different types of heart diseases require specific approaches for management and treatment.

Coronary artery disease (CAD) is at the forefront of heart-related ailments. It's characterized by the narrowing or blockage of the coronary arteries—the vessels supplying blood to the heart. This is caused primarily by the buildup of plaque, a combination of cholesterol, other fats, calcium, and inflammatory cells.

Another significant concern is myocardial infarction, commonly known as a heart attack, which arises when the blood flow to a part of the heart is obstructed, damaging the heart muscle. Immediate attention and treatment are crucial to minimize damage and optimize recovery.

Heart failure, a term that can be misleading, doesn't mean the heart has 'failed' or stopped working. Rather, it describes a condition where the heart doesn't pump blood as efficiently as it should. Managing heart failure involves a comprehensive strategy addressing the underlying cause and supporting heart function with medication, lifestyle changes, and sometimes surgical procedures.

Arrhythmias refer to irregular heartbeats. These can be harmless or life-threatening, depending on the type and severity. Whether it's a heartbeat that's too fast, too slow, or irregular, arrhythmias disrupt the effective pumping action of the heart.

We shouldn't overlook the significance of congenital heart defects either, which are structural problems with the heart present from birth. These range from simple defects with no symptoms to complex abnormalities that cause severe, life-threatening symptoms.

Heart valve diseases involve one or more of the four heart valves not functioning correctly. This can result in the impairment of blood flow through the heart to the rest of the body and can be caused by stenosis, regurgitation, or atresia.

Cardiomyopathy denotes diseases of the heart muscle itself, which can lead to a weakened heart. Different types of cardiomyopathies exist, each with unique causes and treatment requirements. The condition can lead to heart failure and arrhythmias if not managed appropriately.

Pericarditis is inflammation of the pericardium, the sac-like covering of the heart. This can cause sharp chest pain and other symptoms that necessitate medical evaluation and treatment, though in many cases, it's not serious and can improve on its own.

Aortic diseases involve conditions affecting the aorta, the large artery carrying blood from the heart to the rest of the body. An aneurysm or dissection of the aorta can be life-threatening and requires immediate medical attention.

Vascular diseases affect the network of blood vessels outside your heart. These can range from diseases in your arteries, arterioles, veins, and capillaries. Peripheral artery disease, for instance, affects blood flow to the limbs and is a frequent vascular problem.

It's imperative to realize that heart infection, such as endocarditis, is also classified under heart diseases. These infections can damage the heart valves and disrupt normal heart function, requiring aggressive treatment to combat the infection.

Understanding these various conditions is essential in personalizing and fortifying our defenses against heart disease. Each type calls for a distinct approach to prevention, detection, and treatment. We must be mindful that the markers of heart health extend beyond the absence of disease; they also reflect the ability to maintain a heart-strong lifestyle.

Don't let the multiplicity of these conditions overwhelm you. Instead, let it motivate you to be vigilant about your heart health, to arm yourself with knowledge, and to foster habits that shield you from these adversaries. At the same time, embrace the power you have to affect positive change in your heart's well-being through informed choices.

Our journey in battling heart disease requires us to be relentless yet reflective, to make choices that honor the vitality of our hearts. As we press on, let's remember that each stride we take is a choice for our heart's future. Acknowledge the variety and complexity of heart diseases as a challenge to be met with the full force of our determination and the wisdom of careful strategy.

Statistics and Why Men Are at Risk

Heart disease remains the silent killer that shadows men, often without clear symptoms until it's too late. Statistically, men are at a disproportionate risk of heart disease compared to women, with the CDC reporting heart disease as the leading cause of death for men in the United States. This is not just a concern for older adults; young men are also falling prey to this relentless adversary. A confluence of factors such as higher rates of smoking and alcohol use, less likelihood to seek medical care, and societal pressures to ignore pain can lead men down a path to compromised heart health. Understanding these risks and statistics is crucial, as they compel us to confront the reality that many cases of heart disease can be prevented. Through awareness and intervention, we transform these somber statistics into rallying cries for action—stepping stones toward a future where heart health is placed at the forefront of every man's journey to wellness and longevity.

The Impact of Age, Genetics, and Ethnicity

When considering heart health, it's critical to understand that heart disease doesn't exist in a vacuum. Individual factors such as age, genetics, and ethnicity play pivotal roles in shaping one's risk profile for heart disease. Acknowledging the importance of these aspects is fundamental for a comprehensive approach to maintaining heart health.

The passage of time is inescapable, and with it comes the aging process—a key risk factor for heart disease. As men age, the risk of developing cardiovascular issues increases. This is partly due to the natural changes in the heart and blood vessels that occur with age, such as stiffening of the blood vessels and thickening of the heart's walls. Therefore, recognizing that age is more than just a number is essential—it's a factor that demands attention and proactivity in the pursuit of heart health.

But your age does not act alone; it's intertwined with the intricate web of your genetic makeup. Genetics are the framework you're built upon—information passed down from your ancestors that influences how your body functions. Certain genetic markers have been linked to an increased likelihood of heart disease. For males, who may inherit any number of these markers, understanding family history is the key to unlocking the door to proactive personal health measures.

Ethnicity, much like genetics, is an undeniable contributor to heart disease risk. Various ethnic groups show differing patterns of susceptibility to heart disease, which can often be traced back to both genetic predisposition and cultural lifestyle factors. For example, African American men are known to have a higher risk for heart disease compared to their counterparts from other ethnic backgrounds, largely due to higher rates of hypertension and obesity.

Consider the facts: as we drill down into the data, we observe that Hispanics and Latinos are also at heightened risk but often face unique challenges, such as less access to preventative care. Understanding these disparities is not about assigning blame but about informing targeted approaches to heart health that recognize and honor everyone's unique risk factors.

In light of ethnicity and heart disease, we must also address the impact of social determinants of health, including socioeconomic status and access to healthy food and quality healthcare. These directly influence heart health outcomes across different ethnic groups and add yet another layer of complexity to the picture.

While it may seem that your age, genetic code, and ethnic background have dealt you a predetermined hand, the truth is far more empowering: your lifestyle choices can still steer the ship toward healthier shores. Regular screening for heart disease and associated risk factors such as high cholesterol and high blood pressure, particularly in high-risk groups, is a navigation tool you can't afford to ignore.

With advancements in genetic testing, individuals now have access to invaluable information about their personal genetic predispositions to heart disease, information that can guide a preventative approach tailored to one's unique circumstances. It's an ally in the fight against heart disease, illuminating the pathway you should take.

Knowledge of one's genetic makeup should be coupled with mindfulness about how your cultural background may shape your diet and lifestyle choices. Cultural cuisines rich in saturated fats and sodium, for instance, if not modified, might add to your risk factor ledger. It is an invitation to tweak traditions with heart health in mind, without losing the essence of one's heritage.

Another piece of the puzzle is understanding that genetic predisposition doesn't necessarily seal one's fate; genes can be influenced by the environment—namely, your lifestyle choices. Embracing a heart-healthy diet and engaging in regular physical activity can mitigate some inherited risks. This idea is at the heart of the burgeoning field of epigenetics, which studies how behaviors and environment can affect the way genes work.

The effect of age on heart health necessarily links to the importance of life stages. During middle age, one must become vigilant as many heart disease factors often become more pronounced. This is a critical juncture to intercept the trajectory of heart disease with proactive health strategies. Perhaps consider it a rite of passage to a more health-conscious lifestyle.

For older adults, dealing with heart disease may become part of daily life, but that doesn't mean resignation. Even at an advanced age, strategies exist to bolster heart health, ensure quality of life, and even reverse some conditions. It's never too late to start making positive changes.

Focusing on heart health also includes being conscious of how both mental and physical stressors over a lifetime can accumulate and impact the heart. Understanding and managing stress are not just about feeling less pressure—it's about real physiological benefits for your heart, which are crucial regardless of age or genetic background.

In conclusion, while age, genetics, and ethnicity undoubtedly shape the narrative of heart health, they are not the entirety of the story. An informed approach to these factors can illuminate a heart health journey that is proactive, personalized, and ultimately powerful. It's a journey that involves understanding risks, embracing preventative measures, and cultivating a lifestyle that aligns with heart-healthy principles—all with the goal of writing a future that gleams with the promise of longevity and vibrant health.

The conversation around heart health is incomplete without addressing these foundational elements. They are the bedrock upon which you can build a heart-health fortress. The key lies in transforming information into action. When armed with knowledge, nimble strategies, precisely tailored to your individual story, can be masterfully executed. Every informed choice you make is a victory for your heart's wellbeing, and that is a cause for celebration and continued, steadfast commitment.

Chapter 3:
The Warning Signs and Symptoms of Heart Disease

A s we venture deeper into the heart's workings, it's paramount to identify the red flags your body waves when something isn't quite right. Recognizing the signals can be your most potent defense against the sneakiest adversary—heart disease. Chest discomfort is the most classic symptom, but the heart communicates trouble in subtler ways too. Shortness of breath, palpitations, fatigue, and even stomach pain can be the heart's cry for help. Meanwhile, jaw, neck, or back pain, especially if it comes on suddenly, can be silent but dire warnings. Don't ignore the symptoms that may seem trivial—they can escalate quickly. The onset of something as innocuous as a cold sweat or nausea can herald a heart attack or another cardiac event. Ignorance isn't bliss when it comes to your heart. Learn the lexicon of discomfort that your heart uses to alert you, and take these signs seriously to safeguard your health.

Recognizing a Heart Attack

Heart attacks are life-threatening medical emergencies that require immediate attention. By educating ourselves on the warning signs and knowing what to look for, we can take decisive action that could preserve not only the quality of our lives but potentially save them. Of all the information surrounding heart health, recognizing a heart attack is possibly the most crucial.

A heart attack occurs when blood flow to the heart muscle is blocked. It is a pivotal moment when cells within the heart muscle begin to die due to the lack of oxygen. Understanding this mechanism, it's clear why recognizing a heart attack and responding urgently is vital.

One of the first indicators of a heart attack is often chest pain or discomfort. This isn't always the dramatic clutching of the chest seen in movies. It can be a deep ache, a pressure that feels like an elephant sitting on your chest, or a squeezing sensation that can last for a few minutes, or go away and then return. It's imperative to recognize that chest pain can vary greatly from person to person and in intensity.

Other symptoms include discomfort in other areas of the upper body. This can manifest as pain or discomfort in one or both arms, the back, neck, jaw, or stomach. Again, the feeling isn't necessarily sharp or crippling, but it is usually significant enough to cause noticeable discomfort.

Shortness of breath is another warning sign; it could occur before or during the chest discomfort. It might feel like you've just run a sprint, even if you haven't moved. Breathing can become challenging, and you might feel as if you can't catch your breath.

Additional symptoms might include breaking out in a cold sweat, nausea, or lightheadedness. The onset of a heart attack is often associated with a sudden sweat and a feeling that you might pass out. Keep in mind, symptoms might differ between men and women, with women more likely to experience shortness of breath, nausea/vomiting, and back or jaw pain.

Lest we fall into a trap of complacency, it's essential to recognize that heart attacks can occur any time – during vigorous activity or in a state of rest. Even if you're not sure it's a heart attack, any unusual or unexplained symptoms should be checked out immediately.

Another important aspect to remember is that heart attacks can have silent or atypical presentations, particularly in those with diabetes, where nerve damage might dampen the typical pain signals. Silent heart attacks may not have any of the typical signs; instead, they might manifest subtly in the form of fatigue, indigestion, or a general feeling of being unwell.

Some individuals might experience a phenomenon known as 'warning angina'. This is chest pain resulting from exertion that goes away with rest and happens days or weeks before a heart attack. This is the heart's way of sounding the alarm that a more serious event might be near.

If you or someone you know starts to exhibit any of these symptoms, especially if they're combined or persistent, this is a call to immediate action. Don't wait to see if symptoms pass. The sooner a heart attack is recognized and treated, the better the chances of survival and less damage to the heart.

Call emergency services immediately. Many people delay because they're in denial about the symptoms, but time is of the essence. The longer the heart muscle is without oxygen, the greater the damage. Emergency responders can begin treatment as soon as they arrive and are equipped to revive someone if their heart stops.

While waiting for emergency services, if the person is conscious and not allergic, an aspirin can be beneficial as it helps to thin the blood and can slow the progression of a heart attack. It's crucial, though, to always follow the instructions of emergency service operators.

Understanding risk factors are an adjunct component to recognizing a heart attack. High cholesterol, high blood pressure, obesity, diabetes, and a family history of heart disease all increase the likelihood of suffering a heart attack. Knowing your risk can prime you to be more attuned to the signs your body might send.

While heart attacks may seem sudden, they're often the result of long-term heart disease. That's why implementing lifestyle changes, as we will explore in subsequent chapters, is essential. It's more than recovering from a heart event; it's about transforming your life to prevent one from occurring.

Motivation to change can be fueled by understanding the risks and recognizing the signs. It's the power of information that leads to action. Let's be clear: your heart is the life engine of your body. You have the responsibility to keep it healthy and beating strong. Staying informed, vigilant, and proactive is the pathway to heart health. Recognizing a heart attack could be the most crucial knowledge you ever acquire – it is knowledge that could, quite literally, save your life.

In closing this section, it is vital not only to remember these symptoms and warning signs for yourself but to share this lifesaving knowledge with those around you. It's not hyperbole to say that being equipped with this information and the readiness to act swiftly can turn any bystander into a hero. Together, let's be heart attack aware and heart health advocates, not just for our own sakes, but for our families, friends, and communities at large.

Symptoms of Stroke

Embarking on a heart-healthy journey means being equipped with the knowledge to recognize when the body is in trouble. A stroke, often referred to as a "brain attack," challenges heart and brain health alike. In this chapter, we will guide you through the vital signs and signals of a stroke, empowering you to act promptly should one occur.

Identifying a stroke quickly can be the difference between full recovery and long-lasting disability. One of the most recognized tools for spotting stroke symptoms is the acronym F.A.S.T. This stands for Face drooping, Arm weakness, Speech difficulty, and Time to call emergency services. When a stroke strikes, the clock starts ticking, and every second counts.

Face drooping is a clear sign that something may not be right within the brain's pathways. When the muscles on one side of the face fail to receive the proper signals due to brain impairment, that side may sag or fail to respond, signaling a potential stroke. Ask the person to smile; is their smile uneven or lopsided?

Arm weakness or numbness, particularly on one side, is another red flag. Encourage the person experiencing symptoms to raise both arms. Does one arm drift downward, or is it unable to rise at all? This indicates a loss of strength or coordination associated with stroke.

Speech difficulty often presents as slurred or strange-sounding words and can include trouble understanding speech. When the parts of the brain responsible for language are impacted, the simple act of forming coherent sentences can become arduous or even impossible.

Time to call emergency services cannot be overstressed. If someone shows any of these symptoms, even if they disappear, it's imperative to call 911 immediately. Quick response can greatly improve the chances of recovery by reducing the amount of brain damage that occurs.

Beyond the F.A.S.T. criteria, other symptoms can provide early warnings of a stroke. Sudden confusion or trouble understanding simple statements may arise. Unexplained dizziness, loss of balance, or an abrupt severe headache with no known cause are also noteworthy symptoms requiring immediate attention.

Visual disturbances, including sudden trouble seeing in one or both eyes, can signal a stroke. This might manifest as blurred vision, blackened vision, or seeing double. The visual system relies on healthy brain function, and interference from a stroke can hurt visual processing.

Furthermore, a sudden numbness or weakness can occur in the leg, not just the arm or face. Stroke can impact any part of the body, affecting muscle control and sensation. Difficulty walking, stumbling, or a sudden lack of coordination are signs that demand urgent medical care.

A less common but equally important symptom to be aware of is a sudden, severe headache. Unlike headaches associated with tension or sinus issues, a stroke-related headache seems to appear out of nowhere and is often accompanied by other stroke symptoms.

Men should pay special attention to these symptoms, as their likelihood of disregarding physical warning signs can lead to delayed treatment. It's essential to overcome any instinct to "shake it off" or wait for symptoms to resolve on their own.

While these symptoms can be startling, understanding them provides a crucial defence in preserving health and function. Knowledge catalyzes action, and in the context of a stroke, action can mean survival, recovery, and maintaining the quality of life.

It can be helpful to remember that stroke symptoms can vary widely from person to person. Subtle differences in symptom presentation shouldn't be ignored, and any sudden change in neurological function should be treated seriously. Stroke comes unannounced, and that is why constant vigilance is crucial.

In light of these potential warning signs, it's also beneficial to consider the risk factors for stroke that align with those of heart disease — including high blood pressure, smoking, obesity, and diabetes. Management of these conditions not only supports heart health but also reduces the risk of stroke.

Symptoms of a stroke may be fleeting, known as a transient ischemic attack (TIA), often called a "mini-stroke." While the symptoms of a TIA may resolve on their own, this event should not be taken lightly. It's a significant warning sign that a more serious stroke could occur in the future unless intervened upon with appropriate medical treatment and lifestyle changes.

In conclusion, being mindful of stroke symptoms directly supports the health of the heart and brain. This awareness is a powerful tool, and when combined with quick action, it can profoundly alter the outcome of a stroke. Remain attentive to your body's signals, pay heed to these symptoms, and if necessary, act F.A.S.T. to secure the best possible prognosis.

When to Seek Emergency Care

Within our lives, our heart functions tirelessly, often without the acknowledgment or awareness of its ceaseless rhythm. Yet, when our heart signals distress, it's imperative we listen and respond with the urgency this life-sustaining organ deserves. Understanding when to seek emergency care can mean the difference between a full recovery and lasting damage, or even life and death.

One cannot overstate the importance of recognizing the signs that warrant immediate medical attention. Chest pain that persists, is severe, or spreads to the arms, neck, jaw, or back is a red flag that should not be ignored. This type of pain might also come with a pressure or squeezing sensation – a classic symptom of a heart attack.

Breathlessness is another critical symptom demanding swift action. If you find yourself gasping for air or struggling to breathe for no obvious reason, it's time to call for help. This could indicate heart failure, a pulmonary embolism, or even a heart attack. Difficulty breathing while lying down, known as orthopnea, may also be a sign of a failing heart.

An irregular heartbeat, or arrhythmia, that is rapid, fluttering or feels like it's skipping beats can suggest a serious issue. Some arrhythmias may pass without harm, but if accompanied by dizziness, fainting, shortness of breath, or chest discomfort, seek emergency care immediately.

Let's not forget the silent but ominous indicator of lightheadedness or sudden dizziness. This could point to a drop in blood pressure because the heart isn't pumping the way it should. If these symptoms are combined with any other warning signs, it's crucial to get to an emergency room.

Unexplained fatigue or weakness that suddenly hits you can be a harbinger of a cardiac event. Don't dismiss it as merely a bad day, especially if it's intense and out of the ordinary for you. When your body is using energy to fight something potentially harmful, like a heart blockage, fatigue can be your warning system.

Persistent and unexplained coughing that may produce white or pink blood-tinged mucus can signal heart failure. The accumulation of fluid in the lungs, or pulmonary edema, needs immediate attention to prevent a catastrophic outcome.

When cold sweats come out of nowhere, often coupled with other symptoms like chest pain or breathlessness, it's a signal your body is under stress from a potential cardiac crisis. It's a gross understatement to suggest taking it seriously – treat it as the emergency it is.

Nausea or lack of appetite, especially if accompanied by digestive disturbances, can be associated with heart conditions. Although often overlooked, these gastrointestinal symptoms along with the sensation of indigestion could mean your heart is at risk.

Sudden onset of weakness or paralysis in arms or legs, trouble speaking or understanding speech, and face drooping are all indicators of a stroke. Time is brain – every minute matters, so act fast and dial emergency services promptly.

It's worth noting that heart disease symptoms can be subtler in some individuals, and it's vital not to dismiss mild but unusual symptoms, especially if you have underlying risk factors for heart disease. The best course of action is erring on the side of caution.

Be mindful that heart attack symptoms in men can differ from those in women. Men are more likely to experience the classic symptoms, like chest pain, while women may encounter more nuanced symptoms like abdominal pain or extreme fatigue.

Mental preparation is also key in recognizing these symptoms. Having a plan for how to respond to these signs could save crucial minutes. Keep emergency numbers handy, know where your nearest hospital is, and if able, let someone know you're experiencing distress.

The unspoken hero in all of this is prevention. Recognize the power you hold in altering the course of your heart health through lifestyle and dietary changes, as advocated throughout this book. Yet, in moments when prevention gives way to the necessity of urgent care, let nothing hold you back from seeking help.

In times of crisis, recognizing and responding to these warning signs becomes not only a testament to the value you place on your life but a call to action that underscores the importance of heart health awareness. Never hesitate, for it's in our most critical moments that the heart reveals not only its vulnerability but its profound resilience.

Chapter 4:
The Stroke Connection

Engaging with our heart's health without acknowledging the risks and connections to stroke would be to overlook a critical aspect of cardiovascular care. Heart disease and stroke are bound together by a common thread—both arise from compromised vascular health. Understanding this connection begins by grasping that strokes, much like heart attacks, are predicated on the disruption of blood flow, but in the brain rather than the heart. Formulating defensive strategies against this cerebral threat involves a holistic approach, encompassing diet, exercise, and managing risk factors like hypertension and atrial fibrillation. It's imperative to comprehend that, while the risk of stroke escalates with age, it can be combated effectively with preventative measures and lifestyle adjustments. This chapter aims to illuminate the pathways between heart disease and stroke, and most importantly, empower you to reinforce your defenses against this all-too-common accomplice of heart disease.

Understanding Stroke

As we deepen our knowledge on heart health, it's vital to recognize the closely intertwined relationship between heart disease and stroke. A stroke occurs when blood flow to a part of the brain is interrupted or reduced, depriving brain tissue of oxygen and nutrients. Within minutes, brain cells begin to die, which can have lasting effects on one's health or, unfortunately, can even be fatal.

Understanding the various types of strokes is crucial. An ischemic stroke, which is caused by a blockage in an artery leading to the brain, accounts for the majority of stroke cases. A transient ischemic attack, often called a mini-stroke, is caused by a temporary clot and should serve as a serious warning. A hemorrhagic stroke, on the other hand, occurs when a blood vessel in the brain bursts.

Recognizing the symptoms of a stroke can save not only one's quality of life but also their very life itself. Common signs include sudden numbness or weakness in the face, arm, or leg, especially on one side of the body; confusion; trouble speaking or understanding speech; visual disturbances; difficulty walking; dizziness; loss of balance or coordination; and a sudden, severe headache with no known cause. Time is a critical factor, and immediate medical attention can be the difference between recovery and significant disability.

When it comes to heart health, it's important to be aware of the risk factors that make a stroke more likely. Some of these, like family history, age, and ethnicity, can't be changed. However, many stroke risk factors are largely within our control. High blood pressure, high cholesterol, obesity, diabetes, and cardiovascular disease are significant factors that one can manage through lifestyle changes and medication when necessary.

Looking at the causes of stroke provides a compelling reason to focus on heart health. Atherosclerosis, the buildup of plaques in one's arteries, can lead to both heart attacks and stroke. Atrial fibrillation, an irregular heart rhythm, can cause clots that may travel to the brain and induce a stroke. Managing these conditions is a key part of stroke prevention.

Lifestyle changes play a monumental role in reducing the risk of stroke. Smoking cessation, regular physical activity, a balanced diet, moderation in alcohol consumption, and weight management can all contribute to healthier arteries and a healthier heart. The interconnected nature of these lifestyle factors means that improvements in one area can positively affect others, creating a cascade of health benefits.

Knowledge about stroke isn't solely for its prevention—it's also essential for understanding recovery. A stroke can have a variety of long-term impacts, including paralysis, memory loss, difficulty speaking, and emotional challenges. The road to recovery can be a challenging one, with the need for various therapies and support from family, friends, and healthcare professionals.

Preventing a secondary stroke is another critical aspect of the conversation. Those who have experienced a stroke are at higher risk of having another, making it even more important to address all modifiable risk factors and stay vigilant about following treatment plans. Adherence to prescribed medications to manage blood pressure, cholesterol, and blood clotting must be seen as life-sustaining.

Empowerment comes from education. Understanding the relationship between stroke and the body's broader health systems allows individuals to make informed decisions. Regular health screenings, understanding personal health metrics, and the pursuit of medical advice are all proactive steps that can head off potential problems before they manifest as a stroke.

Stroke rehabilitation is a specialized field focusing on relearning skills that a person lost because of brain damage. Rehabilitation can help a person regain independence and improve the quality of life. Support from specialized rehabilitation teams including physio-therapists, occupational therapists, speech-language pathologists, and others, is often fundamental to the recovery process.

Emotionally, experiencing or being at risk for a stroke can be deeply unsettling. Cultivating a mindset of resilience and hope is important. Leveraging a support system, including peer groups for stroke survivors, can provide emotional sustenance and practical advice for living with the changes brought on by a stroke.

Advances in medical technology and treatment approaches offer hope and help reduce the damage caused by strokes. Innovative treatments, such as thrombectomy for certain types of ischemic strokes, may extend the time window for effective intervention, providing a light at the end of a sometimes darkened tunnel.

Finally, partaking in consistent and meaningful conversations with healthcare providers can make a profound difference in both stroke prevention and management. Being transparent about health concerns, symptoms, and family history allows for more accurate assessments and better-personalized care strategies.

Each person's stroke risk profile is as unique as their fingerprints. Therefore, personalized risk assessments are essential. These assessments take into account the complex interplay of genetics, lifestyle, and other factors to provide a comprehensive view of one's risk and create a targeted prevention plan.

In sum, understanding stroke is about being informed, proactive, and resilient. It is through this lens that heart health and stroke prevention converge, creating a foundation for a healthier future. Grasping the intricacies of stroke empowers individuals to take control, actively engage in their well-being, and ultimately forge a path toward a healthier heart and mind.

Prevention and Recovery Strategies

Armed with a deeper understanding of stroke, we pivot towards powerful tactics for its prevention and the pivotal steps to recuperate effectively post-stroke. Establishing a vigilant lifestyle empowered by key preventive measures and deploying timely, targeted recovery strategies can dramatically decrease stroke risk and enhance recovery outcomes. Engaging in regular, dynamic physical activity sharpens cardiovascular resilience, while vigilant monitoring of blood pressure and cholesterol becomes a linchpin in deflecting strokes. Furthermore, a harmonious diet rich in vital nutrients lays a robust foundation to ward off stroke. Should a stroke occur, recovery is catalyzed by an unwavering commitment to rehabilitation, which is not simply a reactionary measure, but a protracted journey of regaining strength, dexterity, and neurological function. The essence of these preventative and recovery strategies rests on the ability to seamlessly fuse them into daily life, crafting a resilient bastion against the tides of stroke and encouraging the body's innate capacity to mend the delicate tapestry of neurons and blood vessels. In the dance between prevention and recovery, every step counts, with each healthful choice sowing seeds for a robust heart and a vigilant, reinvigorated brain.

The Role of Rehabilitation in Stroke Recovery

Rehabilitation is a cornerstone of recovery for men who have suffered a stroke. The journey of healing and adapting post-stroke is critical to regaining strength, abilities, and independence. It's common to wonder about the road ahead, but rehabilitation offers a structured path to reclaim the highest quality of life possible. And yes, while it does entail hard work, the rewards of perseverance can be life-altering.

The initial steps in a rehabilitation program often begin as soon as a patient is stable, sometimes within the first 24 to 48 hours after a stroke. At this stage, the goals of rehabilitation are to prevent complications, minimize impairments, and maximize function. A multidisciplinary team of healthcare professionals crafts a personalized rehabilitation plan, focusing not just on the physical deficits but also on cognitive, emotional, and social aspects of recovery.

Physical therapy stands out as a critical component of post-stroke rehabilitation. It focuses on improving motor skills, strength, and balance. It is normal to encounter frustration as the body may not respond as before the stroke; however, incremental progress with regular physical therapy is a beacon of hope on the road to recovery. Exercise programs are tailored for each individual, taking into account the severity of stroke, general health, and specific impairments.

Occupational therapy is equally integral, as it nurtures the ability to perform daily activities. Therapists support stroke survivors in relearning skills such as dressing, cooking, and bathing, effectively promoting independence. Adaptive strategies and assistive devices may become part of daily routines, paving the way for self-reliance and confidence.

Speech and language therapy addresses difficulties in communication and swallowing, which are common after a stroke. By engaging in language exercises and alternative communication methods, patients can recover the ability to articulate their thoughts and needs, which is fundamental not only for their safety but for their social integration and emotional well-being.

Cognitive retraining is an aspect of stroke rehabilitation that may not be as immediately evident as physical challenges but is no less crucial. Cognitive deficits after stroke can influence memory, attention, and problem-solving skills. Therapists work with survivors to develop new strategies for managing these changes, often incorporating memory aids and structured routines into their daily lives.

Emotional support during this journey is of paramount importance. Psychological counseling and support groups provide avenues for stroke survivors to express their feelings, cope with changes in their lives, and connect with others sharing similar experiences. These outlets assist in overcoming the potential depression and anxiety that can accompany the post-stroke adjustment period.

Nutrition often plays a role in rehabilitation, as proper diet can aid in overall recovery and help manage risk factors for subsequent strokes. Dieticians offer guidance on eating plans that support health and healing, emphasizing whole foods rich in nutrients and low in saturated fats and sodium.

Another core element of stroke rehabilitation is education. Understanding the mechanics of stroke, its effects, risk factors, and prevention strategies empowers patients and their families to take charge of the recovery process and make informed decisions about lifestyle and healthcare.

Transition services are a key facet of stroke rehabilitation, as they focus on the shift from hospital to home care or to another care setting. It is vital that stroke survivors and their caregivers receive training and resources to ensure a safe and supportive home environment.

As recovery progresses, vocational rehabilitation may become relevant for some stroke survivors. Returning to work can boost self-esteem and financial stability but may require adaptive technology or job retraining. Despite potential challenges, reclaiming a role in the workforce is a testament to the progress made in recovery.

Throughout the rehabilitation process, it's crucial to set realistic and achievable goals. Celebrating small victories garners strength and motivation to press onward, remembering that improvement can continue to occur for years post-stroke. It's about valorizing progress over perfection, fostering a mindset of growth and resilience.

Moreover, the role of technology in stroke rehabilitation is evolving rapidly. Innovations such as virtual reality, robotics, and wearable devices offer new opportunities for engaging and effective therapies that can enhance traditional rehabilitation methods.

Finally, it is essential to keep in mind the unique challenges and needs that men may face during stroke rehabilitation. Gender-specific health considerations and the potential impacts on identity and roles within the family and society can require tailored support strategies.

Rehabilitation after a stroke is a journey of transformation that requires dedication, patience, and support. It is a collaborative venture in which survivors, families, and healthcare professionals work in tandem to traverse the complexities of healing. The path ahead might seem daunting, but with each step forward, the realms of possibility expand, exemplifying the human spirit's determination to thrive against the odds.

Chapter 5:
Lifestyle Choices for Heart Health

Embarking on a path to better heart health is a transformative journey that involves a series of intentional choices and changes. In this chapter, we explore critical lifestyle adjustments that can significantly reduce your risk of heart disease and enhance your overall well-being. Optimal heart health goes beyond just diet and exercise; it's about cultivating habits that have a profound impact on your cardiovascular system. You'll learn how saying no to cigarettes is one of the best decisions you can make for your heart, recognizing that smoking cessation is not just beneficial but essential. We'll delve into the management of stress, highlighting its insidious effects on heart health and offering practical strategies to mitigate its impact. Additionally, we'll uncover the often underappreciated role of sleep in maintaining a healthy heart rhythm and restoring your body. By adopting these lifestyle pillars, you are setting the stage for not only a healthier heart but also an improved quality of life that radiates through every aspect of your being.

Quitting Smoking

Embarking on the road to cardiovascular well-being begins with a critical and often challenging step: quitting smoking. Every puff of a cigarette dispatches a cavalcade of toxic substances directly into the bloodstream, wreaking havoc on the cardiovascular system. The evidence is indisputable; smoking is a leading cause of heart disease, yet the journey towards cessation is surmountable when approached with determination and the right support systems.

The path to quitting starts with a compelling vision of a healthier life. Imagine the future free from the shackles of nicotine addiction – a life where every breath is cleaner, and every heartbeat is stronger. It's important to visualize this smoke-free life vividly and often, as this will serve as the lighthouse guiding you through rough waters.

Understanding the health implications of smoking can serve as a powerful motivator. Smoking contributes to atherosclerosis – a buildup of plaque in the arteries that can lead to catastrophic events such as heart attacks and strokes. By discontinuing smoking, you not only halt further damage but the body also begins to repair itself, reducing the risk of heart disease significantly over time.

Setting a quit date is the next logical step. Choose a date not too distant in the future; this helps to establish a concrete goal. Be strategic—the quit date shouldn't be a period of high stress or social gatherings where smoking temptations are abundant. Marking this date on your calendar solidifies your commitment to the decision to quit.

Developing a quit plan is integral to your success. This includes identifying triggers that prompt your smoking habits and establishing strategies to resist or avoid these prompts. Whether it's following meals, during periods of stress, or when in the company of other smokers, planning alternatives for these situations can bolster your resolve to stay smoke-free.

Seek out support. This can come from family, friends, or a community of individuals with the shared goal of quitting. Many find encouragement in support groups or smoking cessation programs. Bring your inner circle into this journey; their support can be critical during moments of weakness.

Consider nicotine replacement therapy (NRT) or medication approved by healthcare professionals. These are designed to reduce withdrawal symptoms and the urge to smoke. NRT options like patches, gum, lozenges, inhalers, or nasal sprays can be part of your arsenal in combating cravings.

Behavioral strategies bring another dimension to your quit plan. Techniques such as deep-breathing exercises, mindfulness meditation, or physical activity can help manage the stress and anxiety that often accompany quitting smoking. Reprogramming your responses to stress without reliance on nicotine will be a pillar of your success.

Physical activity is not only a distraction from cravings but also boosts your overall health. Just a short walk can alleviate the urge to smoke and at the same time, enhance your cardiovascular health. As your lungs heal and your body regenerates, you'll find increasing energy levels and higher fitness potential, reinforcing your commitment to remain smoke-free.

While the initial phase of quitting is challenging, ensure you recognize and celebrate milestones. Each smoke-free day, week, or month is an achievement that brings you closer to a heart-healthy life. Rewards can be simple but enjoyable, like a movie night or a small purchase as a reminder of your progress and the money saved from buying cigarettes.

Prepare for setbacks but don't let them derail your efforts. Most people don't successfully quit on their first attempt, and that's okay. Every attempt to quit smoking, even if it doesn't last, brings you closer to the ultimate goal. Learn from past relapses; they can teach invaluable lessons about triggers and strategies that require adjustment.

Eliminate all smoking reminders from your environment. Get rid of cigarettes, ashtrays, and lighters. Clean your home and car to remove the smell of smoke. A clean environment reinforces your new identity as a non-smoker and helps to eliminate cues that might tempt you to light up.

As your journey to quit smoking advances, keep in mind the long-term benefits for your heart. Within a year of quitting, the risk of heart disease drops to about half that of a smoker – an impetus to persist. In nearly 15 years, your risk of coronary heart disease could be akin to that of a person who's never smoked.

Quitting smoking is the cornerstone of protecting your heart from further damage. It's a formidable challenge, but it's one that unleashes a cascade of positive changes for your heart's health. Embrace this process as an opportunity to cultivate resilience, demonstrate self-care, and ultimately, transform your life.

It's important to surround yourself with positive influences and information that reinforce your choice to quit smoking. Educate yourself further on the dangers of smoking, and frequently remind yourself why you're quitting. This approach aligns your mind with your heart's health, creating a synergy that propels you forward, past temptation and into a smoke-free existence.

Finally, never lose sight of why you embarked on this journey. Your heart, the steadfast organ that powers life, deserves the best care you can offer. Quitting smoking is not simply a lifestyle change; it is a profound act of self-preservation that echoes the deepest respect for your body and the life you wish to lead. Embrace this change with enthusiasm and see it not as a sacrifice, but as the path to rediscover the vibrancy and longevity that your heart, and you, truly deserve.

Managing Stress

When contemplating heart health, stress management can't be overstated. It's an integral part of maintaining a healthy lifestyle and is as crucial as a balanced diet or exercise. Chronic stress can wreak havoc on your body, posing serious harm to your heart. Therefore, mastering the art of stress management is not only beneficial for your mental well-being but is also imperative for your physical health.

Understanding the link between stress and your heart starts with the release of stress hormones like adrenaline and cortisol. These increase your heart rate and blood pressure, preparing your body for a "fight or flight" response. In short bursts, this is completely normal; but if your stress response doesn't switch off, the long-term effects can be detrimental to your heart.

So, how can one deal with stress effectively? The first step is recognizing the symptoms of stress, which can be more subtle than one might expect. Symptoms can manifest as irritability, sleeping problems, changes in appetite, and even physical symptoms like headaches or stomach issues. Acknowledging these as signs of stress is the starting point of managing them.

Mindfulness and meditation have shown great promise in stress reduction. These practices involve focusing on the present moment and accepting it without judgement. By incorporating mindfulness into your daily routine, even for just a few minutes, you can dramatically lower stress levels and reduce your risk of heart disease.

Physical activity is another potent stress reliever. Exercise not only improves physical health but also boosts endorphins, which are natural mood lifters. It's not necessary to engage in strenuous workouts; even gentle walking, yoga, or cycling can help ease stress.

Building a strong support network is also crucial for stress management. Connecting with friends, family, or support groups can provide emotional comfort and advice on dealing with stressors. Isolation can exacerbate stress, so maintaining social ties is a key component of a heart-healthy lifestyle.

Time management can significantly reduce stress levels. Many of us feel overwhelmed by our to-do lists, but planning your day, setting priorities, and delegating tasks can help manage the burden. Learning to say no to additional responsibilities can also prevent overloading yourself with more than you can handle.

Practicing relaxation techniques, such as deep breathing exercises, progressive muscle relaxation, or visualization, can help release tension in the body and lower stress hormone levels. These techniques can be performed anywhere and require only a few minutes to make a difference.

Another important aspect is to ensure you get adequate sleep. Sleep deprivation can exacerbate your stress levels, creating a vicious cycle. Establishing a routine that promotes good sleep habits is not only beneficial to manage stress but also vital for heart health.

Diet plays a significant role in managing stress. Consuming a diet rich in fruits, vegetables, whole grains, and lean proteins can provide high levels of nutrients that support physical health and help in countering stress. Avoiding excess caffeine and sugar is also wise, as they can increase tension.

Learning how to manage your emotions is as important as managing externals stresses. Sometimes, cognitive behavioral therapy or other forms of counseling can be invaluable in this regard, teaching you how to change negative thought patterns that contribute to your stress.

For those moments when stress is unavoidable, it's important to have coping strategies in place. This could be as simple as taking a few deep breaths, stepping outside for a breath of fresh air, or finding humor in a stressful situation.

It's sometimes necessary to seek professional help if stress becomes overwhelming and you find it hard to cope. Healthcare providers can offer a range of therapies and stress management programs tailored to your needs.

Don't underestimate the importance of hobbies and leisure activities in stress reduction. Engaging in activities you enjoy can be a powerful antidote to stress and can bring much needed balance to your life.

Finally, be patient with yourself. Stress management is a skill that takes time to develop. Be kind to yourself as you learn and apply these new techniques and remember that managing stress is an ongoing process that contributes greatly to the health of your heart.

By incorporating these strategies into your life, you'll be well on your way to minimizing stress's toll on your heart. Embrace each day as an opportunity to enhance your heart health, and allow every choice you make to be a step towards a calmer, more balanced existence.

The Importance of Sleep

When journeying toward a heart-healthy lifestyle, sleep often emerges as an unsung hero. This foundational pillar of health wields an astonishing influence on the heart's wellbeing. Forging a relationship with our pillows that prioritizes quality and quantity of sleep is a powerful yet often overlooked strategy in buttressing heart health.

Embracing the quietude of night, allowing the body to recuperate from daily stresses, isn't just a luxury—it's a necessity. Adequate sleep has been linked to reduced inflammation, a factor closely tied to heart disease. During sleep, the body engages in vital processes of repair and rejuvenation, which includes moderating blood pressure and heart rate.

Yet, the path to slumber is beleaguered for many. The pressures of modern life can push sleep down the ladder of priorities, leading to a deficit that can have profound effects. Shortchanged rest doesn't just lead to next-day fatigue; it incrementally contributes to a more insidious erosion of cardiovascular health.

Understand that sleeping patterns influence metabolism and weight—an important consideration for heart health. Sleep deprivation can disrupt the balance of hunger hormones, such as ghrelin and leptin, often leading to increased appetite and potentially contributing to obesity, a key risk factor for heart disease.

Moreover, the quality of sleep matters. Obstructive sleep apnea, a condition characterized by pauses in breathing during sleep, is associated with hypertension, arrhythmias, and an increased risk of heart disease. It's essential to be mindful of sleep quality, and to consult healthcare providers if there's a suspicion of such sleep disorders.

Interestingly, not just any sleep will do. Diving into the rejuvenative depths of slumber means achieving enough deep sleep, that stage in which the heart rate and breathing slow down, and the body achieves its most restorative work. Prioritizing a sleep environment that promotes uninterrupted sleep is just as essential as setting aside the hours to rest.

Stress and sleep maintain a bidirectional relationship. High stress levels can decimate sleep quality, and insufficient sleep can increase stress and its negative impacts on the heart. It's crucial to manage stress effectively to ensure it doesn't encroach on the sanctity of sleep.

In the pursuit of restful nights, we must take heed of our daily rituals. Regular exercise, as mentioned in earlier chapters, not only strengthens the heart but can enhance sleep quality. However, timing matters. Engaging in vigorous physical activity too close to bedtime can be counterproductive, as it may delay sleep onset.

Diet choices, too, play a starring role in the nighttime drama. A diet high in saturated fats and sugars can thwart efforts to fall asleep quickly and sustain a deep sleep state. Conversely, a heart-healthy diet that includes nutrients like magnesium and omega-3 fatty acids can be conducive to better sleep.

Sleep should be respected as a crucial player in the game of heart health. Setting a consistent sleep schedule is a strategic move toward establishing good sleep hygiene, bolstering heart health with every stroke of the circadian rhythm.

As we explore the myriad of choices for maintaining a healthy heart, don't underestimate the power of the night. Sleep is not merely a passive state; it is an active, dynamic process that shores up the defenses of our cardiovascular system.

So heed this call to action: assess your sleep, improve it if necessary, and make it an unshakable part of your daily routine. Treasure your sleep as a rejuvenative elixir for your heart, for it's in these quiet hours of repose that your body works tirelessly to maintain the rhythm of life.

Let's consider, for a moment, the relationship between sleep and the medications many heart patients take. Some medications can interfere with sleep architecture and quality. If you're noticing disturbances in your sleep pattern, speak with a healthcare provider about potential medication adjustments or interventions to mitigate these effects.

An embrace of sleep's importance is a commitment to holistic health — a recognition that wellness weaves through every hour of the day and night. By championing sleep as a fundamental component of heart health, we create an environment in which our hearts can beat strongly and resiliently for years to come. So tonight, as every night, let sleep be a sanctuary for your heart.

Chapter 6:
Nutrition for a Healthy Heart

Transitioning from a focus on the pivotal role of lifestyle in heart health, we venture into the transformative power of nutrition in cultivating a heart-strong existence. A well-curated diet isn't just about restriction; it's the cornerstone of cardiovascular vitality. With an emphasis on whole, unprocessed foods, we'll explore the symphony of nutrients that supports cardiac function and discourages disease. Choosing the right fats to champion heart health, integrating fiber-rich foods that champion arterial cleanliness, and selecting quality proteins that bolster cell repair are more than dietary changes—they are acts of reverence for the heart's ceaseless labor. We'll dissect the myths surrounding heart-healthy diets and elucidate the pathways through which balanced nutrition can beat back the spectres of hypertension and atherosclerosis, leaving you equipped to craft a daily menu that celebrates and sustains your heart's rhythm. This chapter isn't just a list of dos and don'ts; it's an invitation to savor the medley of flavors that nature offers, fostering a peace treaty with food to embolden your heart against the ailments that challenge it.

Heart-Healthy Diet Basics

Transforming your diet is a powerful way to protect your heart. It isn't just about restricting yourself; it's about embracing a diverse range of foods that can heal, strengthen, and energize your body. A heart-healthy diet is rich in nutrients, fiber, and healthy fats, and it's crucial to prioritize these while minimizing the intake of sodium, added sugars, and trans fats.

Eating for a healthy heart begins with understanding the building blocks of your food. Carbohydrates, found in grains, fruits, and vegetables, should be consumed in their whole and unprocessed forms. Whole grains, like oats and quinoa, can help manage cholesterol levels, while fruits and vegetables are full of antioxidants that support heart function.

Proteins are essential for repairing and building tissues in the body. When choosing protein sources, opt for lean meats like poultry and fish, which are lower in saturated fat. Plant-based proteins such as lentils, beans, and tofu are also excellent choices, offering fiber and heart-healthy nutrients without the added fats found in some animal proteins.

Fats play a significant role as well. While it's important to limit saturated fats, which are found in high-fat dairy and red meat, healthy fats are vital for heart health. These include monounsaturated fats found in olive oil and avocados, and omega-3 fatty acids present in fish such as salmon and mackerel.

Limiting sodium intake is another key aspect of a heart-healthy diet. High sodium levels can lead to hypertension, a major risk factor for heart disease. Instead of salt, flavor your meals with a variety of herbs and spices, which can also offer additional health benefits.

It's also important to stay hydrated. Water is the best choice for maintaining good hydration levels without added sugars or artificial sweeteners. Replace sugary drinks with water or unsweetened herbal teas to reduce your calorie intake and decrease your risk of weight gain and diabetes.

Beyond these basics, portion control plays a role in a heart-healthy diet. Eating too much of even the healthiest foods can lead to weight gain and stress on the heart. Learn to listen to your body's hunger and fullness cues and try to eat smaller, more frequent meals to manage appetite and energy levels.

Incorporating a wide variety of fruits and vegetables into your diet is not only beneficial for heart health but also for the overall nutritional value they bring. These superfoods are packed with vitamins, minerals, and fiber, all of which are critical for maintaining a healthy heart and body.

Being mindful of the quality of the food you eat is as important as what you eat. Processed foods often contain hidden sugars, fats, and sodium, so focusing on fresh, whole foods will ensure you're not unintentionally consuming these harmful ingredients.

When it comes to cooking for heart health, methods matter. Grilling, baking, steaming, and sautéing with a small amount of healthy oil can enhance flavors without the need for added salts or fats. This approach preserves the nutrients in the food and prevents the creation of harmful byproducts that can occur with frying.

Alcohol consumption should be moderated, as excessive drinking can lead to an increase in blood pressure and can contribute to irregular heart rhythms. For men, this typically means no more than two drinks per day. Remember that a "drink" is defined as 12 ounces of beer, 5 ounces of wine, or 1.5 ounces of spirits.

Understanding food labels is crucial. Start by looking at the serving size and then check for crucial information like total fats, cholesterol, sodium, and added sugars. This knowledge will empower you to make informed choices and avoid foods that may seem healthy at first glance but are actually detrimental to your heart health.

Meal planning can help establish a pattern of healthy eating. Taking the time to create a weekly menu, prepare ingredients in advance, and ensure that a variety of nutrients are included can make it easier to stay on track with your heart-healthy diet.

Lastly, don't forget that a heart-healthy diet is not just about the individual ingredients or nutrients—it's about the overall pattern of eating. Strive for balance and variety, and remember that making small, steady changes to your diet can lead to significant improvements in your heart health over time.

Embrace the journey towards a heart-healthy lifestyle with enthusiasm and optimism. Your heart is the engine of your life, and by nurturing it with the right foods, you'll be setting the pace for a future that's richer not just in years, but in vitality and joy.

Foods to Eat and Avoid

Embarking on the journey towards a robust heart necessitates a discerning palate—one that welcomes heart-friendly foods while shunning those that undermine cardiovascular vitality. To fortify your heart, infuse your diet with verdant vegetables, brimming with vitamins, fiber, and essential nutrients. Luxuriate in the simplicity of whole grains; their integral role in managing blood pressure is indisputable. Lean toward proteins that echo the rhythm of a healthy heart, such as fish rich in omega-3 fatty acids, legumes, and skinless poultry. Let's not forget the blissful crunch of nuts and the virtuousness of seeds, both allies in this noble fight. However, the landscape of nutrition also harbors villainous elements that you're wise to avoid. Processed foods, sirens of convenience, are laden with sodium, undercutting your heart's health with every tempting bite. Trans and saturated fats, found in red meat and full-fat dairy, plot silently against arterial wellbeing. And finally, the seductive sweetness of added sugars—found in sodas, desserts, and more—can lead to weight gain and metabolic turmoil. Be vigilant; choose sustenance that aligns with your heart's deepest yearnings for health and longevity.

The Role of Supplements in Heart Health

In the pursuit of optimal heart health, a balanced diet stands as the cornerstone. Yet, even the most meticulously planned meals can fall short of delivering all the essential nutrients necessary for heart health. Here we explore how supplementation can serve as a strategic ally in fortifying one's nutrition landscape and bolstering heart health.

Navigating through the world of supplements can be overwhelming, given the abundance of options available. It's important to understand that supplements are not a cure-all but can complement a heart-healthy diet and lifestyle. Let's delve into specific supplements that have been associated with cardiovascular benefits and learn how they can integrate into a heart-focused wellness plan.

Omega-3 fatty acids, omnipresent in fish oil supplements, are widely acclaimed for their anti-inflammatory properties and potential to reduce the risk of heart disease. These essential fats can't be produced by the body and must be obtained either through diet or supplementation. By lowering triglyceride levels and potentially stabilizing heart rhythm, omega-3 supplements become a topic of discussion for those looking to support their cardiac health.

Another supplement of note is Coenzyme Q10 (CoQ10), a substance akin to a vitamin, found naturally in the body and key to energy production. As levels can decline with age and certain medications, such as statins used to lower cholesterol, supplementation may help replenish CoQ10 to aid in maintaining a healthy heart muscle.

Following CoQ10, Magnesium emerges as an essential mineral with a role in over 300 biochemical reactions in the body, including the regulation of heart rhythm and arterial health. Keeping in mind that magnesium deficiency is not uncommon, supplements may help meet daily requirements to promote cardiovascular wellness.

When it comes to managing cholesterol, Niacin, a form of Vitamin B3, makes an appearance. Niacin has been used to increase high-density lipoprotein (HDL), the "good" cholesterol, which helps to transport fat away from arteries and reduce the risk of atherosclerosis. However, it's important to approach Niacin supplementation cautiously, as high doses can lead to adverse effects.

Taking a step towards the realm of antioxidants, supplements containing Vitamin E have been studied for their potential to protect against the oxidation of LDL cholesterol, thought to play a role in the development of heart disease. Despite early enthusiasm, recent studies suggest a more nuanced view, emphasizing a balanced approach to antioxidant supplementation.

Fiber supplements also come into play as a valuable addition to a heart-healthy dietary regimen. Soluble fiber, in particular, can help reduce absorption of cholesterol into the bloodstream, complementing dietary sources such as oats, beans, and fruits.

Another supplement gaining attention is L-arginine, an amino acid which is believed to help relax blood vessels and improve blood flow. Although our body typically produces enough L-arginine, supplemental doses may provide additional heart benefits for certain individuals.

Garlic supplements also warrant examination, as they have been recognized for their potential effects on blood pressure and cholesterol levels. While culinary usage of garlic is widespread, concentrated doses in supplement form may amplify these cardioprotective attributes.

Moving beyond individual nutrients, there are proprietary blends and specific formulations that claim to support heart health. It's crucial to approach such products with a discerning eye and consult a healthcare professional before integrating them into your routine.

Caution is paramount when considering any supplement. It is essential to contemplate potential interactions with medications or other supplements, as well as recognize that some supplements may have side effects or lead to excess intake of certain nutrients.

Ensuring quality is another significant concern. Supplements are not regulated to the extent that pharmaceuticals are, so it's vital to select products from reputable manufacturers that adhere to high standards of quality and testing.

Bringing the discussion into the personal domain, the use of supplements should be tailored to individual needs. Factors like dietary restrictions, health conditions, and specific nutrient deficiencies will influence the supplementation strategy most beneficial for you.

Prioritizing a dialogue with healthcare providers is indispensable. A professional can offer guidance on which supplements are evidence-based and suitable for your unique health profile, helping to integrate them safely and effectively into your heart health regimen.

In conclusion, supplements can play a supportive role in heart health. They are not a substitute for a nutritious diet or healthy lifestyle but can act as valuable instruments in your heart-health toolbox. With informed choices and professional guidance, supplements can contribute to a comprehensive strategy for cardiovascular wellness.

Chapter 7:
Exercise Your Way to a Stronger Heart

If you're looking for a powerful ally in the fight for heart health, lace-up those sneakers, because exercise is your trusty partner on this journey. Engaging in regular physical activity is akin to fortifying your heart with armor, and the benefits reach far and wide, from improving blood pressure to boosting your cholesterol profile. But it's not just about warding off heart disease; exercise also empowers you with increased energy, better sleep, and an enhanced sense of well-being. In this chapter, we'll dive into how you can tap into the transformative power of movement, debunk myths that may be holding you back, and devise a personalized exercise plan that's not only effective but also enjoyable and sustainable. You'll learn how to tune into your body's signals and pace yourself for optimal gains, ensuring your heart gets stronger day by day, and with every beat. Let's harness the vitality that physical fitness offers and embark on a path where every step, every lift, and every stretch moves you closer to a heart that doesn't just beat, it thrives.

Benefits of Regular Exercise

Immersing ourselves in the rhythm of a healthier lifestyle, we find the core of well-being in the simplicity of movement. Regular exercise, a pinnacle of proactive health maintenance, casts a wide net of benefits for heart health, especially for those pondering the significance of every heartbeat. By intertwining physical activity into the fabric of daily life, the heart not only gains strength but also the resilience required to pump vitality throughout our bodies.

The heart, a muscular powerhouse, thrives on the challenges presented by regular physical exertion. Like any muscle in need of conditioning, the heart responds to exercise by enhancing its pumping capacity and efficiency. Endurance activities such as brisk walking, cycling, or swimming encourage the heart to pump blood more effectively, reducing the workload on this vital organ over time.

One significant benefit of regular exercise is the ability to wage war against coronary artery disease. Physical activity promotes the development of new blood vessels, a process known as angiogenesis, ensuring a richer supply of blood to heart tissue. This cultivates an environment where the heart can endure the possible disruptions caused by blockages in arteries.

Beyond the mechanics of blood flow, exercise plays a pivotal role in blood pressure regulation. Incorporating routine exercise can lower blood pressure, a notable adversary in heart disease, and reduce the strain on arterial walls. The resulting ease in vascular tension serves to fortify the body's network of vessels, promoting lasting heart health.

Let's not overlook cholesterol – a familiar term in the lexicon of heart health. Exercise helps modify the types of cholesterol in the body, raising high-density lipoprotein (HDL) or the 'good' cholesterol while diminishing low-density lipoprotein (LDL) or 'bad' cholesterol levels. This balance is critical in mitigating the risk of atherosclerosis and subsequent heart complications.

Diving deeper into the metabolic aspects, regular exercise boosts the body's ability to metabolize glucose. Enhancing this capability not only supports overall energy levels but plays a preventive role in the development of type 2 diabetes, a condition that often walks hand-in-hand with heart disease.

Weight management is another cornerstone. Exercise burns calories, aids in controlling appetite, and shifts the body composition towards a higher ratio of muscle to fat. A healthy weight lessens the heart's burdens, empowering it to serve its purpose without the added strain imposed by excess body mass.

While we focus on physical transformations, it's paramount to recognize the mental fortitude gleaned from regular exercise. Physical activity releases endorphins, the body's feel-good neurotransmitters, which can elevate mood and alleviate symptoms of depression and anxiety, often associated with chronic heart conditions.

The anti-inflammatory effects of exercise whisper another promise for heart health. Chronic inflammation — a silent assailant of cardiovascular wellness — is countered by the anti-inflammatory response elicited by regular physical activity. This can be instrumental in the prevention of heart disease and stroke.

A lesser-known but equally significant benefit is the improvement in sleep quality. Regular exercise can help in falling asleep faster, deepening sleep phases, and reducing the incidence of sleep disorders such as insomnia, all of which have a symbiotic relationship with heart health.

Exercise also helps in cultivating an intimate awareness of one's body and its signals. This heightened sense of self can lead to early detection of potential heart issues, prompting timely medical consultation. It's like learning to interpret a language spoken silently by the body.

For those with existing heart disease, structured exercise can act as a rehabilitative force. Cardiac rehabilitation programs often include tailored exercise routines that can aid in recovery and improve the quality of life post a heart event.

Increased circulation due to exercise also contributes to a more robust immune system. A vigilant immune system not only quickens recovery from illness but also protects against future cardiac events by mitigating potential infections that can affect heart health.

Moreover, the commitment to regular exercise often leads to a cascade of positive lifestyle choices. It's not uncommon to see dietary improvements, tobacco cessation, and better stress management in the wake of an established exercise routine. It's a holistic approach where one good habit begets another, and the heart reaps the benefits.

Lastly, the societal component of exercise — whether in a group setting or part of a community event — nurtures social connections and support networks. These relationships contribute to emotional well-being and provide a mutual encouragement system that is essential for maintaining a heart-healthy lifestyle.

In embracing the advantages of regular exercise, the promise of a stronger heart is not merely a hope, but an attainable reality. Each movement, each elevated beat, echoes a dedication to heart health that deepens with every step, cycle, or swim. The power to sculpt a resilient heart lies within the resolve to move, to endure, and to thrive.

Creating a Personalized Exercise Plan

Embarking on the journey to a stronger heart requires a map that's uniquely yours; a plan that caters to your current health status, your goals, and the activities you enjoy. Imagine crafting an exercise regimen that not only bolsters your heart health but one that you're excited to follow. Start by consulting with your healthcare provider to set safe, realistic goals considering your heart condition. Think of exercises that fit your lifestyle: if you're someone who loves the outdoors, brisk walking or cycling might be your gateway to cardiac fitness. For those who prefer the privacy of their home, resistance bands or body-weight exercises could be the cornerstone of your plan. Remember, consistency is key, so slot your workouts into your schedule like any other vital appointment. And don't forget to integrate flexibility and balance activities; these, too, play a critical role in your heart health. With dedication and a personalized approach, you're not just working out; you're building a robust, healthier heart, one beat at a time.

Staying Motivated for Long-Term Success

This is perhaps one of the most challenging aspects when it comes to maintaining heart health, particularly after a diagnosis of heart disease or in the pursuit of preventive care. The journey to a healthier heart isn't just a matter of making a few simple changes; it's about embedding these changes deep into the fabric of your daily life. This requires an unfaltering commitment to your wellness goals and the ability to keep pushing even when the road gets tough.

Motivation is deeply personal and often based on intrinsic values and goals. Think about what your healthy heart means to you. Is it playing ball with your kids? Is it traveling the world without the fear of a heart attack? Or is it simply enjoying your golden years with vigor and vitality? Keeping your 'why' close to your mind can fuel your willpower on days when it seems easier just to slip back into old habits.

Setting realistic goals is the cornerstone of any successful health regimen. Small, achievable milestones can create a sense of accomplishment that continuously propels you forward. Want to lower your cholesterol level? Start with a small goal, perhaps reducing it by a certain percentage in three months. After you've hit that first target, set another. Celebrate these wins, no matter how small, and let them be the lighthouse guiding you through the fog of occasional disheartenment.

Community plays a crucial role as well. This could be a support group for individuals managing heart disease, a gym buddy, or a family member committed to making dietary changes with you. This network can provide encouragement, hold you accountable, and offer practical advice when facing obstacles. Even on days when your personal resolve might waver, knowing that others are invested in your success can be an intensely powerful motivator.

Progress is not always visible, and plateaus are common. When this happens, shift your focus away from the scale or the numbers on your blood pressure monitor. Reflect on how your lifestyle changes have improved other areas of your life. Maybe you're sleeping better, your moods have improved, or you have more energy to partake in activities you love. These signs indicate that your hard work is paying off, beyond just the traditional markers of health.

Education is also a potent tool for maintaining motivation. Learning about heart disease, its risks, and how your efforts are making a difference can boost your resolve to stick with healthy lifestyle changes. Dive into books, documentaries, or even reputable online resources that shed light on the benefits of a heart-healthy lifestyle and the risks of neglecting your heart's well-being.

Adapting to change can't be a punishment; it must be a new way of living that you genuinely enjoy. Incorporate activities you love into your exercise regimen. If the gym isn't your scene, consider hiking, biking, or swimming. These activities do not punish your body but rather celebrate its capabilities and the improvements you're creating within it.

Feedback and reflection are integral to staying motivated. Keep a journal to record your experiences, emotions, and progress. On tougher days, looking back at how far you've come can be incredibly uplifting. Taking this time to introspect also allows you to re-evaluate strategies that might not be working and pivot accordingly.

Eating habits can often be the hardest to change, given their cultural and emotional connections. Approach this as an opportunity to learn and experiment with new recipes and flavors. This can help relieve the monotony of a 'diet' and instead transform it into a culinary adventure that benefits both your taste buds and your heart.

It's important to integrate flexibility into your routine. Life is unpredicatble, and rigid structures can break under the weight of unforeseen circumstances. If you miss a workout or enjoy a birthday cake, don't let it derail your entire plan. Accept it, enjoy the moment, and return to your routine without guilt.

Consider professional guidance to maintain momentum. A dietitian or a personal trainer specifically versed in heart health can provide personalized advice and adjustments to keep you on track. This type of tailored support can often address the unique challenges that come with individual health conditions.

Acknowledge and prepare for setbacks as a natural part of the journey. Not every day will be perfect, and unexpected health issues might arise. It's not the setback itself but how you respond to it that matters. Reinforcing your strategies during these times can not only help you bounce back but also strengthen your resilience.

Visual cues can keep your motivation tangible. Whether it's a photo of loved ones you're working hard to stay healthy for, or a chart on the fridge tracking your cholesterol levels—having visual reminders in your everyday life can reinforce your goals and why you set them in the first place.

Lastly, remember to be kind to yourself. Transformation won't happen overnight, and that's okay. The heart is a muscle that gains strength not from sporadic bursts of energy but from continuous, committed care. Patience is vital, as is recognizing that this is a lifelong journey of nurturing the engine that sustains you.

In summary, staying motivated for long-term success in heart health can be challenging, but it's definitely achievable with the right mindset and tools. Keep your 'why' in mind, set realistic goals, lean on your community, educate yourself, enjoy the process, be flexible, seek professional guidance, prepare for setbacks, use visual cues, and treat yourself with compassion. Your journey towards a healthier heart is one of the most important investments you'll ever make—embrace it with perseverance and optimism.

Chapter 8:
Tackling Obesity and Weight Management

Embarking on the journey to manage weight is a critical step in fortifying heart health. The ties that bind obesity to heart disease are unambiguous, with excess weight acting as both a catalyst for and a predecessor to cardiac issues. Addressing this challenge invites a deliberation of energy, commitment, and a sturdy strategy for weight loss that respects the body's needs while setting attainable targets. In this chapter, we'll navigate the complexities of shedding pounds in a manner that's safe and profound, with an emphasis on long-term transformation rather than ephemeral fixes. We'll equip you with the tools to intelligently calibrate your food intake, amplify your metabolic fire, and align your mental resolve with your physical aspirations. It's about understanding the risks associated with weight, but also recognizing the power you hold to reshape your health destiny. As we dissect the mechanics of successful weight management, remember that each step forward is a stride towards a heart-resilient future.

The Link Between Weight and Heart Health

Engaging our awareness in the relationship between weight and heart health invites a transformative journey towards optimal well-being. Excess weight stands as a significant contributor to numerous cardiovascular diseases – a fact supported by a robust body of scientific evidence. This nexus is not mere correlation but rather one of causality, where additional pounds can lead to substantial heart risks.

The pathology begins with how excess weight, particularly around the abdomen, fosters systemic inflammation. This inflammation acts as a catalyst, damaging blood vessels and leading to atherosclerosis—a condition characterized by the hardening and narrowing of arteries. These changes within the circulatory system can precipitate heart attacks, heart failure, and other life-threatening events.

Another link in the chain is hypertension, or high blood pressure, which can manifest due to increased body weight. The heart has to work harder to pump blood through additional body mass, which in turn increases the force against your artery walls, magnifying the risk of heart disease. For heart health, keeping blood pressure in check is non-negotiable.

Moreover, excessive weight often accompanies abnormalities in cholesterol levels, including hikes in harmful LDL cholesterol and dips in protective HDL cholesterol—each a harbinger for coronary heart disease. The balance of lipids in our bloodstream significantly influences the integrity of our vascular system, where the correct equilibrium sustains heart health, and any disproportion threatens it.

Striving towards a healthy weight should not be enshrouded in aesthetic goals alone, but anchored in the quest to mitigate metabolic disorders like insulin resistance and type 2 diabetes. These conditions bolster cardiovascular diseases, often existing as intertwined phenomena with obesity, leading to a compounded threat to heart health.

The impact of weight on cardiovascular health is not limited to adults; emerging research is casting light on how childhood obesity plants the seeds for adult heart disease. Therefore, addressing weight issues early on can serve as preventative medicine, forestalling the potential for heart-related maladies in later life.

To harness this knowledge is to empower oneself to make informed choices. It's about understanding that each meal, each activity, each decision we make can tip the scales towards a healthier heart. Managing weight is not merely about vanity; it's about vitality— it's about living a life with an empowered heart that beats strong not just for today, but for all the tomorrows ahead.

Yet acknowledging the bridge between weight and heart health is but the first step on this path. We need to understand that weight loss can be a pivotal strategy to reduce the strain on the heart and enhance its function. The heart can recover some of its vigor once the load it carries is lightened, thus rectifying some of the damage inflicted by excess weight.

Bariatric surgery outcomes often cast a spotlight on the dramatic improvements in cardiovascular health post-weight loss, indicating that when weight decreases, heart health exponentially improves. However, we emphasize that surgical routes are but one option; many can achieve substantial heart health benefits through non-surgical, lifestyle-centered means of weight management.

Starting with a comprehensive approach that includes a heart-healthy diet, regular physical activity, stress reduction, and proper sleep hygiene holds the promise of not only shedding pounds but rejuvenating the heart. In this landscape, we recalibrate our lifestyle by committing to daily choices that elevate our heart's well-being.

Steadfast resolve, coupled with patience, is imperative in this endeavor. Quick fixes and fad diets may show immediate results but seldom lead to sustained heart health. The target is a lifetime of balance and wellness – seeking weight loss that brings along enduring heart health benefits.

It can't be overstated how important it is to enlist professional guidance in this journey. A healthcare provider can offer personalized advice, taking into account individual health status, preferences, and goals. A tailored plan can ensure safety, efficacy, and sustainability when endeavoring to improve both weight and heart health.

Embracing technology can augment our efforts. Advances in wearables and health apps offer unprecedented ability to track physical activity, dietary intake, and even stress levels—each a piece of the larger puzzle of weight and heart health management. They serve as virtual allies, empowering us to remain on course towards our objectives.

Finally, it is a collective journey. The support of family, friends, and communities creates an environment conducive to positive changes. They are the cheerleaders in one's corner, the sounding boards for frustration, and the companions in celebrating the triumphs—big and small—on the road to a heart-healthy weight.

In summation, by drawing on the inexorable link between weight and heart health, we can harness a powerful lever to transform our cardiac well-being. This section will cast light on implementing effective strategies for weight management, aligning with the heart's needs, and paving the way for a fuller, more vibrant life. It's about taking control, one heartbeat and one step at a time.

Strategies for Losing Weight Safely

Embarking on a journey to shed excess pounds is a commendable step towards enhancing heart health, but it's vital to approach weight loss with a strategy grounded in safety and sustainability. Begin with a well-balanced diet rich in whole foods, incorporating a variety of fruits, vegetables, lean proteins, and whole grains, while limiting processed foods and sugar-laden snacks that can sabotage weight-loss efforts. Regular physical activity is a cornerstone of healthy weight management; aim for a mix of cardiovascular exercises and strength training to boost metabolism and build muscle. Remember, moderation is key; drastic calorie cuts can do more harm than good.

Partner with a healthcare provider to tailor a weight loss plan that aligns with your individual health needs and monitor your progress. Water intake should be ample, as hydration is crucial for optimal body function and curbing unnecessary hunger pangs. Lastly, ensure that sleep is not compromised; ample rest is often underrated yet critical in the weight loss equation, as it helps regulate hunger hormones and repair the body. By implementing these strategies with patience and persistence, you'll be on a path to a healthier, more fulfilling life, underpinned by the notion that each step forward is a victory in its own right.

Tracking Progress and Setting Realistic Goals

Embarking on the journey to better health, especially after grappling with weight-related issues, requires dedication, patience, and importantly, a structured approach. It's essential to track progress as you venture forward. However, tracking isn't just about stepping on the scale; it involves a comprehensive look at various markers of health and adjusting your targets to stay aligned with your personal health goals.

Begin by setting realistic, measurable goals. Realistic goals are those that consider your current lifestyle, your medical background, and your personal capacities. They should stretch you but still be attainable. For instance, a goal to lose a certain amount of weight is good, but consider how much time it will require based on a healthy rate of weight loss, which is typically 1 to 2 pounds per week.

Measuring progress can take many forms beyond weight. It can include body measurements such as waist circumference, body fat percentage, or even changes in clothing sizes. These metrics can be more telling than weight alone, since muscle is denser than fat and weight can fluctuate with water retention. Remember to celebrate the non-scale victories that occur along the way.

Maintain a progress journal or use an app to log your daily diet, exercise routines, and any obstacles you encounter. Having a written record provides tangible proof of your progress and encourages continued adherence to your plan. It also enables you to identify patterns or triggers that might be slowing your progress, so you can adapt your strategy as needed.

Setting incremental milestones within your larger goals can keep your motivation high. For someone with heart disease, a milestone could be as simple as walking a certain number of steps without getting winded or cooking heart-healthy meals three times a week. Reward yourself for meeting these smaller goals, but avoid rewards that counteract your efforts, like high-calorie treats.

Stay patient and kind with yourself. There will be setbacks, and weight loss plateaus are a natural part of the process. During these times, focus on what you've already achieved and the health benefits you're experiencing, even if they're not completely evident on the outside.

Involve your healthcare team in your goal-setting and progress tracking. Regular check-ups can provide professional insights into your health status. Your doctor, dietician, or trainer can help tweak your plan, ensuring you stay on the safest and most effective path towards your health goals.

Consider also tracking your blood work results, such as cholesterol levels and blood pressure, as these are crucial indicators of heart health. By observing how these numbers change over time, you can get a more scientific measure of the benefits your lifestyle changes are providing.

Understanding your body's responses to various foods and activities is crucial. You may notice that some exercises are more enjoyable or some foods leave you feeling more energized. Use this information to make your health journey more personalized and effective.

Remember, progress is progress, no matter how small. It can be tempting to compare your journey with others', but every individual's body is unique. What works for one person may not work for another, so focus on your own path and the strides you're making.

Managing stress, which is a significant contributor to heart health issues, should be included in your progress tracking. Notice if stress management techniques are helping lower your blood pressure or improve your heart rate variability. Including these in your progress markers gives a holistic view of your overall wellbeing.

Staying hydrated and getting enough sleep are two aspects that often get overlooked when tracking health progress. Yet, they are vital components of a heart-healthy lifestyle. Observe and record your sleep patterns and water intake as these can have significant effects on your energy levels and heart health.

Lastly, be adaptable. Life happens, and there may be days or weeks where you can't stick to your plan as rigidly as you'd like to. Use your progress tracking system to accommodate for these life events and adapt your goals accordingly without feeling like you've taken a step back. It's about forward movement, however gradual that may be.

Tracking progress and setting realistic goals are foundational to managing obesity and weight, but they also play a significant role in the broader context of managing heart disease. By staying committed to this process and continually adapting to new insights and changes in your health status, you lay the groundwork for a heart-healthy future. Every step taken, every healthier choice made, contributes to a stronger, more resilient heart and a higher quality of life.

Through diligence, perseverance, and a clear understanding of where you stand and where you're heading, you can turn the tide against heart disease. Remember, this is your path, one that you carve out step by step with every informed choice and every goal achieved.

Chapter 9:
Managing Blood Pressure and Cholesterol

Embarking on the journey of heart health, we've explored the foundations of heart anatomy, unearthed the dangers of heart disease, and delved into the lifelines of prevention through lifestyle and diet. Now, we arrive at the vital crossroads of managing two key indicators of cardiovascular health: blood pressure and cholesterol. With precision and understanding, it's possible to steer these markers toward optimal levels, much like navigating a ship through calm waters. Recognizing the significance of the numbers that define your blood pressure, you're equipped to interpret what they reveal about your heart's workload and the health of your blood vessels. It's more than just numbers; it's about understanding the silent language of your body as it whispers hints of your overall well-being. Similarly, a nuanced understanding of cholesterol's role reveals that not all cholesterol is a foe; it's a delicate balance between the good and the bad, which can either protect or endanger your heart's vitality. Strategies for managing these crucial indicators don't just rest on the shoulders of medication but are deeply rooted in the power of lifestyle choices. Empowering yourself with knowledge, you can tweak your diet, refine your exercise regime, and realign your life's daily rhythms to foster an environment where blood pressure and cholesterol levels are not adversaries but allies in your quest for a robust heart.

Understanding Blood Pressure Numbers

In our endeavor to navigate the complex terrain of heart health, a crucial metric stands out for its undeniable significance: blood pressure. Comprehending blood pressure numbers isn't just about reading values; it represents insight into the very essence of our well-being. Blood pressure readings serve as a beacon, guiding us through the fog of medical ambiguity to the shores of informed decision-making.

Blood pressure is denoted by two distinct numbers, a symbiotic pair providing a glimpse into the ebb and flow of our circulatory system. The upper number, known as the systolic blood pressure, reflects the pressure exerted upon the arteries' walls when the heart muscle contracts. It's the drumbeat your heart sounds with each forceful contraction, propelling life-giving blood throughout your body.

Conversely, the lower number, the diastolic blood pressure, speaks of rest - it measures the pressure in the arteries when the heart rests between beats. It whispers of the moments of calm, a serene interval as the heart gathers itself for the next surge.

A standard blood pressure reading might come across as "120 over 80" or 120/80 mmHg. These figures are more than mere numbers; they are critical indicators of your cardiovascular harmony. The optimal range for health leans toward the lower threshold of normalcy, with figures such as 120/80 mmHg being the gold standard for many adults.

The elevation of these numbers is where caution must be exercised. High blood pressure, or hypertension, is often dubbed the "silent killer". It whispers negligible symptoms or none at all, yet its impact can be catastrophic, orchestrating a coup within the body that can lead to heart attacks, strokes, and kidney failure.

Understanding the thresholds of blood pressure is crucial. Any systolic figure between 120 to 129 mmHg with a diastolic pressure below 80 mmHg nudges you into the elevated category, a yellow light signaling the need for lifestyle adjustments and vigilance.

Hypertension stage 1 is characterized by systolic numbers between 130 to 139 or diastolic numbers between 80 to 89 mmHg. This stage warrants more than attention—it's a call to action, perhaps a lifestyle recalibration or medication for some.

Hypertension stage 2 climbs the ladder with systolic numbers of 140 mmHg or higher or diastolic numbers of 90 mmHg or higher. This stage accentuates the seriousness of the situation, often necessitating immediate medical intervention.

A hypertensive crisis, where systolic pressure soars above 180 mmHg and/or the diastolic pressure exceeds 120 mmHg, is a health emergency. It dredges up the urgency for immediate medical care to prevent a catastrophic cardiovascular event.

It isn't merely about knowing these numbers but understanding that behind each digit lies an intricate interaction between your heart and the vast network of arteries. Each heart pump and each moment of rest contributes to these readings, which when combined, paint a portrait of your vascular health.

To stay ahead of the curve, regular monitoring is essential. A blood pressure cuff isn't just a band of fabric and air; it's a tool of empowerment. With it, you capture a real-time snapshot of your circulatory system's state, enabling proactive management of your heart health.

Lifestyle modifications are the cornerstone of maintaining or improving these vital statistics. Engaging in regular physical activity grounds the heart in strength, adopting a heart-healthy diet serves as nourishment for vitality, and managing stress works to still the internal storms that may disrupt your cardiovascular equilibrium.

However, for some, lifestyle adjustments may not suffice. Medication in coordination with the guidance of healthcare professionals can steer blood pressures back to safer waters. It's the collaborative effort between patient and doctor that often charts the course for success.

Remember, these numbers are not static; they are dynamic markers that can be influenced by actions, behaviors, and sometimes, genetic predisposition. It bears repeating – monitoring these figures is not an optional part of your journey. It is as integral as the blood coursing through your veins.

Your commitment to understanding and acting on your blood pressure numbers is testament to the value you place on your heart's health. It's an ongoing dialogue between you and your body, a conversation that can lead to proactive changes, fostering a future of improved wellness and vitality. As you journey through these pages, know that each step taken towards comprehending and managing your blood pressure is a stride toward a more heart-healthy existence.

Strategies for Managing High Cholesterol

Mastery over cholesterol levels is a pillar of heart health that can't be ignored. It's about understanding the subtle dance between lifestyle choices and the biological outcomes that follow. Embarking on this journey requires a tactical approach to dietary intakes, such as embracing foods rich in omega-3 fatty acids and soluble fiber, while saying a firm 'no' to trans fats and foods with high levels of saturated fat. Consider this the choreography that protects your heart. Physical activity isn't just for aesthetics; it's a potent weapon in your arsenal for boosting 'good' HDL cholesterol, which helps to sweep away the 'bad' LDL cholesterol from your arteries. Additionally, maintaining a healthy weight isn't just beneficial for your self-image; it's a critical movement towards optimal cholesterol levels. Pharmaceutically, when lifestyle maneuvers can't rein in those stubborn cholesterol figures, statins or other lipid-lowering meds might be the reinforcements needed. However, it's essential to carry out this concerted effort under the watchful guidance of your healthcare provider, ensuring every step forward is a stride towards vitality. Remember, this isn't about quick fixes but a long-term commitment to a heart-harmonious lifestyle.

The Importance of Regular Health Screenings

Embarking on the journey of maintaining your heart health is akin to navigating a complex terrain—it requires vigilance, proactive steps, and regular checkpoints. This is where the importance of regular health screenings becomes not just beneficial, but essential. Regular health screenings serve as pivotal moments in your journey to heart health, offering you snapshots of where you stand and how your lifestyle changes are impacting your risk factors for heart disease.

Health screenings are not merely about prevention; they are about empowerment. Knowledge of your body's current state can inform your decisions, enabling you to adjust your lifestyle in the most effective manner. These screenings seek out the silent issues that might otherwise go unnoticed until they manifest as urgent health crises. Conditions like hypertension and high cholesterol can lurk without clear symptoms, yet they are leading risk factors for heart disease and stroke.

Screenings also offer baseline data which is vital for tracking progress. When changes are made to your diet or exercise routine, ongoing screenings can show you the fruits of your efforts in real time. This feedback loop can serve as a powerful motivator, highlighting the positive impact of healthy choices and allowing you to course-correct early if necessary.

Consider the screenings as a tool for personalized healthcare. Each individual's risks and health status differ, and thus, the screenings you undertake might vary from another person's. Your family history, age, current health status, and even occupation can influence the types of screenings most pertinent to you. One size does not fit all in the realm of preventative health. In this sense, think of health screenings as a tailored suit, meticulously fitting to your specific needs and altering with time and changes in your health and lifestyle.

Timing is a critical factor in the effectiveness of health screenings. There is a schedule to adhere to, often based on guidelines set by medical organizations, which recommends at what age and how frequently certain screenings should occur. For men with a predisposition to heart disease, these intervals may be shorter, emphasizing the need for closer monitoring.

Let's discuss the financial aspect too. Preventative health care through regular screenings can also serve as a cost-saving measure. By catching potential issues early, management and intervention can prevent more serious, and often more costly, health problems down the line. Consider them an investment in your future well-being and financial health.

In the context of heart health, screenings often focus on blood pressure, cholesterol levels, body mass index (BMI), and blood sugar levels—each a significant indicator of your cardiovascular health. These metrics can reveal the underlying conditions that often contribute to heart disease, such as hypertension, dyslipidemia, obesity, and diabetes. By keeping a watchful eye on these parameters, you're able to take immediate and meaningful action.

It's also worth acknowledging the emotional aspect of health screenings. Getting screened can provoke anxiety, but it's important to remember that they are a proactive step in safeguarding your health. Turning the anxious energy into a more positive and productive force can help you embrace screenings as an opportunity to ensure your longevity and vitality.

Moreover, regular screenings can play a pivotal role in familial health. If you have a family, consider that your diligence in staying healthy sets an example, influencing your loved ones to prioritize their health as well. Communicate openly about the benefits and empower them to join you in regular check-ups.

The dialogue created between you and your healthcare provider during these screenings is invaluable. It's an opportunity for you to be heard, to express concerns, and to ask questions. It enables a deeper level of partnership in managing your health, where your healthcare provider can tailor advice and interventions to your unique situation. This two-way communication is a cornerstone of effective health management.

Screenings are also a cornerstone in the fight against the silent progression of heart disease. Insights gathered can reveal trends, triggering early interventions before a potential heart event occurs. Remember that in the arena of heart health, being proactive is infinitely better than being reactive. A proactive approach can preserve not only the quality of life but life itself.

Health screenings dovetail seamlessly with lifestyle modifications. As you adjust your diet, increase your physical activity, and make other beneficial changes, screening results provide tangible evidence of how these strategies are improving your heart health. They bridge the gap between daily actions and long-term outcomes, showing you the real-time impact of your decisions.

Ultimately, regular health screenings illuminate the path to heart health. They are a fundamental part of a larger strategy that includes diet, exercise, stress management, and other lifestyle choices. They stand as a testament to the belief that the power to change your health destiny is in your hands. By embracing regular health screenings, you're taking control—making informed decisions, adjusting your course when necessary, and celebrating victories along the way.

Maintaining a heart-healthy lifestyle is a dynamic process, a conscious evolution where regular health screenings are your compass. They're an integral aspect of a committed approach to wellness, guiding you through the intricate dynamics of heart health. So, approach your health screenings with respect, anticipation, and a readiness to use the knowledge gained to fuel your journey towards robust cardiovascular health. Your heart, and the lives intertwined with yours, deserves nothing less.

Chapter 10:
Understanding and Managing Diabetes

As we've journeyed through the intricacies of heart health, we've tackled how our lifestyle choices and nutrition significantly impact our well-being. Now we delve into a topic that intertwines closely with heart health: diabetes. This chapter strips down the complexity of diabetes, a condition that can't be overlooked when discussing heart disease, as it doubles the risk for cardiovascular complications. Gaining control over diabetes isn't just about managing blood sugar levels—it's about embracing holistic lifestyle changes that fortify your heart against future adversities. We'll dissect the art of balancing daily activities with dietary considerations and medication adherence, all tailored to reinforce your heart. With every page, you'll gain more clarity and control, equipping you with the tools to not just manage, but thrive, despite diabetes, thus shielding your heart from its potential onslaught.

Diabetes and Heart Disease Connection

As we delve into the intricate relationship between diabetes and heart disease, it's essential to recognize the substantial impact that one has on the other. For those managing diabetes, understanding this connection can be the light guiding you to a healthier heart and a more vibrant life.

Diabetes affects individuals by impairing the body's ability to manage blood sugar levels. Over time, chronically elevated blood sugar can lead to a host of complications, one of the most severe being heart disease—the leading cause of death among people with diabetes.

The correlation between diabetes and heart disease is multifaceted. High blood sugar levels can damage blood vessels and the nerves that control your heart. People with diabetes are also more likely to have other conditions that increase the risk of heart disease, such as high blood pressure and abnormal cholesterol levels.

In essence, the presence of diabetes can significantly elevate the risk of developing atherosclerosis—a condition that hardens and narrows the arteries. Atherosclerosis is like a thief in the night, stealthily advancing and setting the stage for heart attacks, strokes, and other cardiovascular issues.

Let's speak candidly about insulin resistance, often present in people with type 2 diabetes. It's not just a signal of blood sugar trouble; it's a red flag for heart health. Insulin resistance means your body's response to insulin is weakened, necessitating more insulin to manage blood sugar levels. High levels of insulin can be problematic because they encourage the body to hold onto sodium, which increases blood pressure—a pivotal risk factor for heart disease.

Moreover, diabetes can lead to changes in the composition and function of the blood, making clots more likely to form. These clots are traitors in the bloodstream, potentially blocking blood flow and leading to heart attacks or strokes.

Understanding the association between diabetes and heart disease is empowering. It illuminates a path for intervention and prevention, emphasizing the importance of managing blood sugar levels to safeguard the heart.

A diabetes diagnosis doesn't spell inevitable heart trouble. Instead, it is a clarion call to embrace lifestyle changes that can fortify heart health. This resonance carries a message of hope and action—modifying your diet, incorporating regular exercise, and adhering to medications can all work in concert to protect your heart from the menace of diabetes.

Nutrition, undeniably, plays a pivotal role. By opting for a diet rich in fruits, vegetables, lean proteins, and whole grains while reducing the intake of processed and high-fat foods, you can exert a profound influence on both your blood sugar and heart health. This is the harmonious dance between diet and well-being, where every good choice fuels the heart's rhythm.

Physical activity is also paramount—it encourages the body to use insulin more efficiently, thus helping to moderate blood sugar levels. With every step taken, every lift, and every stretch, you are warding off the complications associated with diabetes and bolstering your heart's strength and resilience.

Consistent monitoring of blood sugar levels is a foundational aspect of managing diabetes with the heart in mind. Precision here is not just about numbers; it's about understanding your body's responses and adjusting your lifestyle and treatment as necessary.

It's crucial to acknowledge that while lifestyle adjustments are powerful, medication may also play an essential role in managing diabetes and protecting the heart. Medications can help control blood glucose, blood pressure, and cholesterol levels. Collaboration with healthcare professionals is key in tailoring a regimen that harmonizes with your unique health needs.

Don't underestimate the psychological whispers that urge you toward wellness. The motivation to persist with these lifestyle choices is not merely for the day at hand but for a future where heart and health thrive. Resilience in the face of diabetes is not just surviving—it's about prospering, with a heart beating strong.

In grasping the connection between diabetes and heart disease, you become equipped to navigate the complexities of these health conditions. With the right knowledge and tools, not only can you manage diabetes, but you can also embark on the journey towards a healthier, more inspired life with a heart that's shielded by your informed, proactive choices.

As this voyage continues, let the unity of heart and health be your compass, with each beat affirming life and each controlled blood sugar reading steering you towards calm seas. The heart, resilient and steadfast, can triumph over the challenges presented by diabetes, and it is within this balance that hope and health coalesce into a symphony of wellness for a life rich in vitality and fulfillment.

In the next chapters, we'll explore lifestyle management for diabetics and delve deeper into monitoring and medication compliance. But, remember, with each step forward, you are not only managing diabetes - you are reclaiming command of your heart's destiny.

Lifestyle Management for Diabetics

Lifestyle management for those with diabetes isn't just about monitoring blood sugar levels; it's a full-scale commitment to transforming daily habits to safeguard your heart. Integrating a balanced, nutritious diet rich in fiber and low in added sugars can make a significant difference, maintaining not just stable glycemic levels, but also supporting overall cardiovascular health. Physical activity is equally critical; finding enjoyable ways to move more throughout the day can help manage weight and reduce insulin resistance. A step as simple as replacing sedentary activities with brisk walks can have far-reaching benefits for your heart. Stress, an often-overlooked factor, can impact glucose control and heart health. Embracing techniques such as mindfulness or yoga can help mitigate stress-related spikes in blood sugar and blood pressure. Prioritizing good sleep hygiene is also essential, as inadequate rest can impede your body's ability to regulate hormones and recover. Remember, managing diabetes isn't just about reacting to symptoms; it's about proactively cultivating a lifestyle that supports your heart's health and vitality, establishing a routine that champions wellness at every turn.

Monitoring and Medication Compliance

As you navigate the intricacies of managing diabetes in conjunction with heart disease, monitoring your health and ensuring medication compliance are pivotal steps in the journey. A comprehensive approach to health care, which embraces diligent tracking and management of your blood glucose levels, cholesterol, and blood pressure, forms the cornerstone of both prevention and treatment of heart complications. This section is focused on empowering you to confidently take control of these aspects of your daily routine.

To begin, let's look at the basics of medication compliance. Adherence to prescribed medication is often the heartbeat of managing diabetes and its related cardiovascular risks. Missing doses or not taking medications as directed can lead to suboptimal blood sugar control, which over time can cause serious heart-related complications. Your medication regimen is a tool, meticulously designed to help maintain the delicate balance within your body's systems.

But how do you keep track? The answer lies in creating a system. Whether it's a digital reminder on your smartphone, a pillbox organizer, or a written record in a journal, establish a routine that integrates medication times seamlessly into your daily life. Remain consistent with this routine, and soon it will become second nature. Moreover, ensure you understand each medication's purpose and the crucial role it plays in protecting your heart.

Let's not overlook the importance of monitoring blood glucose levels. Regularly checking your blood sugar provides immediate feedback on the effectiveness of your diet, exercise, and medicine. It also alerts you to potential problems so you can take action before they progress. Invest in a reliable glucose meter, and learn how to use it accurately. Record these readings to discuss with your healthcare provider, facilitating conversations about potential adjustments for optimal control.

Your healthcare team is your ally; be open to discussing any challenges you encounter with medication side effects or the complexities of daily glucose monitoring. They can offer alternative solutions or adjustments to fit your needs and lifestyle. Your honest communication is vital to tailor your treatment plan for success.

Education is also a powerful tool in managing your condition. Understanding the 'why' behind your medication and monitoring routines can motivate you to remain compliant. Utilizing resources provided by healthcare practitioners or credible online information can shed light on the effectiveness and importance of each aspect of your treatment.

Moreover, ensure you stay current with your prescriptions. Running out of medication can lead to gaps in your treatment, so it is advisable to set up a system that alerts you to request refills with ample time. Many pharmacies offer automatic refill programs, and some even provide home delivery services, which can mitigate the risk of noncompliance due to lack of medication.

It is also essential to recognize that lifestyle modifications can and should complement your medication regime. A heart-healthy diet and regular exercise can significantly improve diabetes control and reduce heart disease risk factors. Your commitment to these areas can lead to a reduced need for medications and result in a more potent, synergistic protective effect on your heart health.

Now, what about when you travel or face disruptions to your routine? Have a plan in place for these occasions. It might be a travel pill case, setting alarms at different times due to time zone changes, or having a written medical plan. Predicting these changes and preparing for them ensures continuity in medication compliance and health monitoring.

Remember that your journey with heart health and diabetes is unique to you. Individual variations in metabolism and how your body responds to medication necessitate a customized approach. Working closely with your healthcare provider to adjust medications based on your specific needs and responses ensures the most effective management of your condition.

Fostering a support network can also be beneficial. Whether it's family, friends, or a heart health support group, having others who encourage and assist you with your medication and monitoring regimes can make a substantial difference. They can provide both emotional support and practical assistance when you need it most.

In case you face financial difficulties accessing medications or testing supplies, be proactive. Numerous patient assistance programs are available, offering help for those who qualify. Don't hesitate to explore these options and discuss them with your healthcare provider.

Lastly, celebrate your successes along the way. Every time you maintain your medication regimen, every heart-healthy choice, every successful glucose reading, is a victory worth acknowledging. These achievements reflect your commitment to your heart health and overall well-being.

Monitoring and medication compliance are integral parts of managing diabetes and heart disease. Embrace these practices with determination. By doing so, you're building a foundation for a healthier heart and a fulfilled life. Your heart is at the helm, beating strongly, as you take charge and navigate towards wellness with knowledge, discipline, and resolve.

Chapter 11:
Alcohol, Drugs, and Heart Health

Continuing our journey towards a robust heart, it's crucial to confront the contentious relationship between substance use and cardiac wellness. While moderate alcohol consumption has been touted in some circles for its potential heart benefits, the key lies in understanding that moderation is a slippery slope, and excessive indulgence can cascade into a myriad of heart health issues including hypertension, arrhythmias, and an increased risk for cardiomyopathy. On the flip side, the perilous impact of recreational drugs extends far beyond their immediate intoxicating effects, posing a serious threat to cardiovascular function. From cocaine's adrenaline surge that burdens the heart with excessive demand to the insidious erosion of cardiac tissue by opioids, each substance carries a hidden dagger aimed at the very core of our circulatory system. For those entangled in the grip of substance abuse, acknowledging the problem is a vital first step; seeking help is not a sign of weakness but a courageous act of self-preservation. It is essential to navigate out of these treacherous waters with a support system that can guide you back to the safe harbors of health and longevity, ensuring your heart's rhythm beats in harmony with a life full of vitality.

The Effects of Alcohol on the Heart

When discussing the intricate relationship between alcohol and heart health, it's essential to navigate through the complexities with care. For many, the occasional glass of wine may seem benign, but the overall impact of alcohol on the heart is far from straightforward. This section explores the nuanced ways in which alcohol can influence heart function, dissecting the evidence to empower and inspire informed decisions for those striving to protect their heart health.

Firstly, let's address the proverbial elephant in the room - the belief that moderate alcohol consumption may provide cardiovascular benefits. While some studies have suggested that light to moderate drinking, particularly red wine due to antioxidants such as resveratrol, can have a protective effect on the heart, it's a fine line between moderate consumption and excessive intake which can have deleterious effects. This has led to a contentious debate within the medical community about the net effect of alcohol on heart health.

Delving deeper, we find that the heart isn't just a simple pump; it's a complex organ that can be affected by alcohol in several ways. Alcohol can have an immediate impact on your heart rate, causing it to beat faster. This is often referred to as "holiday heart syndrome," a term that underscores the fact that even non-habitual drinkers can experience atrial fibrillation (a type of irregular heartbeat) after episodes of binge drinking.

For individuals with a history of arrhythmias or other heart conditions, this temporary increase in heart rate and irregular rhythm can exacerbate existing problems, potentially leading to more severe health issues. In these cases, the risks associated with alcohol consumption eclipse any potential benefits.

Chronic alcohol consumption is also linked to cardiomyopathy, a disease of the heart muscle that leads to its enlargement and a disorganized pumping structure. Over time, the heart becomes inefficient at pumping blood, which could ultimately progress to heart failure - a serious condition where the heart can't meet the body's blood flow requirements.

We must also consider alcohol's contribution to hypertension. While you might feel relaxed after a couple of drinks, alcohol actually raises blood pressure, thereby increasing the strain on your heart. Persistently high blood pressure demands that the heart work harder to circulate blood, potentially leading to hypertrophy of the heart muscle, which is a risk factor for heart failure and stroke.

Furthermore, alcohol can influence the lipid profile in the bloodstream. Although moderate consumption has been associated with increases in 'good' HDL cholesterol, heavy drinking can lead to the elevation of triglycerides - a type of fat found in your blood that, at high levels, can increase the risk of heart disease.

Here's an indisputable fact: alcohol contains calories. Excessive consumption contributes to the development of obesity. Weight gain, particularly around the abdomen, is a significant risk factor for heart disease and other health issues such as diabetes, which itself can damage the heart and blood vessels over time.

In addition, the intersection of alcohol and heart medication deserves attention. Alcohol can either enhance or inhibit the effects of various heart medications, which can dangerously lower or wildly fluctuate blood pressure levels, potentially leading to a stroke.

It's not just physical interactions we need to consider. Alcohol can also impact decision-making and lifestyle choices, leading to poor nutrition and reduced physical activity. The domino effect of these choices can further undermine heart health and counteract any potential benefits of moderate alcohol consumption.

In light of these insights, it is evident that moderation is key in alcohol consumption, especially for those with pre-existing heart conditions or risk factors for heart disease. The advice can't just stop at a generic call for moderation; rather, it should be personalized, taking into account one's overall health, lifestyle, and risk factors.

For those who choose not to abstain completely, it's paramount to understand and adhere to what is considered moderate - which for men is up to two drinks per day. Remember, 'drink' sizes are standardized, and consuming larger quantities under the guise of moderation is a common pitfall.

Eliminating alcohol, on the other hand, altogether offers a clear way to reduce many of the described risks. For some, this may sound daunting or unnecessary, but for individuals with heart disease or those at high risk, the benefits of giving up alcohol can be substantial and far-reaching.

As much as we strive to improve heart health through positive actions and interventions, it's equally important to be aware of the elements that can derail our efforts. Alcohol, while legally and culturally pervasive, is one such element that must be managed with careful consideration of the potential heart health ramifications.

So as you move forward on your journey toward optimal heart health, take a moment to reflect on the role alcohol plays in your life. Consult with healthcare professionals, assess your personal health goals and risks, and choose a path that leads to a stronger, healthier heart. You're not simply seeking to avoid heart disease; you're working to foster a life of wellness, vitality, and longevity, where every choice counts towards a more vibrant and fulfilling life.

The Dangers of Recreational Drug Use

The journey to optimal heart health can be fraught with challenges, and the role of recreational drug use is a topic that warrants focused attention. The allure of such substances may be strong, but the toll they take on the cardiovascular system is often grave and multifaceted. Illicit drugs, ranging from stimulants like cocaine and amphetamines to opioids and new synthetic compounds, can have immediate and long-standing effects on heart function. Some substances accelerate the heart rate and increase blood pressure, leading to arrhythmias or a heart attack, particularly dangerous in individuals with existing heart conditions. Opiates, on the other hand, may depress breathing to the point of causing hypoxia, harming not only the brain but the heart as well. Recreational drug use also contributes to a cascade of inflammatory reactions and potential clot formation—catalysts for stroke and heart failure. Considering the silent and cumulative damage these drugs can inflict, making the choice to avoid recreational drug use isn't just a lifestyle preference; it's a life-preserving commitment. Your heart's resilience is a testament to your body's extraordinary potential to recover and renew—but only when provided with a conducive environment for healing and strength.

Seeking Help for Substance Abuse

The journey toward heart health is multifaceted, requiring not just physical but also emotional and psychological fortitude. An often-overlooked obstacle in this journey is the specter of substance abuse, which can significantly set back progress for those with heart disease. Acknowledging that one needs help is an act of bravery and the first step toward recovery.

Substance abuse, whether it involves alcohol, prescription medication, or recreational drugs, poses a severe risk to heart health. These substances can lead to an array of cardiovascular complications—hypertension, arrhythmias, and even heart attacks. Beyond the immediate physical dangers, there is a web of psychological and social factors that must also be addressed.

For individuals who face the rigors of substance dependence, understanding that help is available—and effective—is vital. Recovery programs abound, yet choosing the appropriate one is contingent upon the severity of the addiction, the substance in question, and the support systems in place. Specialized professional help, tailored to address the complex relationship between addiction and heart disease, is a precious resource.

Detoxification is often the initial phase of treatment, and it should be undertaken with medical supervision. Withdrawal can be perilous, sometimes leading to dire cardiovascular events. It is crucial to have a healthcare provider guide this stage, ensuring safety and managing any acute medical issues that arise.

Following detox, rehabilitation programs offer structured support. These programs help to unravel the psychological ties to addiction through therapy, while also reinforcing the development of healthier coping mechanisms. They are designed to provide a stable foundation upon which a substance-free life can be built.

For many, recovery is a long-term process that extends beyond a stay in rehab. Outpatient programs and support groups serve as the scaffolding for a sustained recovery, offering regular check-ins and peer support. Support groups, such as those offered by Alcoholics Anonymous or Narcotics Anonymous, can offer a lifeline to someone struggling to maintain their sobriety.

Moreover, for individuals with heart disease, specialized care teams that include cardiologists, dietitians, exercise physiologists, and mental health professionals can integrate substance abuse treatment into a broader heart health strategy. This intersectional approach acknowledges the intricate nature of recovery and heart disease management.

Mental health treatment plays a critical role in the recovery process. Substance abuse and conditions such as depression and anxiety are often entwined. Addressing mental health can strengthen one's capacity to maintain sobriety and manage heart health. Cognitive-behavioral therapy and other forms of counseling can be particularly effective.

For those with a dual diagnosis—a concurrent mental health condition and substance abuse disorder—integrated treatment that targets both issues simultaneously is essential. Separating heart health from mental health and substance recovery is no longer an acceptable approach in modern healthcare. Treatments that address the holistic needs of the individual have proven to be more effective.

Medical intervention may also be necessary, depending on the individual's condition. Medications can help manage cravings and other withdrawal symptoms and should be considered as part of a comprehensive treatment plan. They must be prescribed judiciously, taking into account potential interactions with other medications for heart disease.

Family involvement can also act as an anchoring force in recovery. Substance abuse can strain personal relationships, yet a strong support network is a cornerstone of successful outcomes. Families need to be equipped with the knowledge and tools to support their loved ones effectively without enabling addictive behavior.

Another component of recovery is lifestyle modification. Integrating into daily life the heart-healthy practices outlined in earlier chapters—balanced nutrition, regular exercise, stress management— can bolster one's ability to stay substance-free. A lifestyle supporting heart health is antithetical to one of substance dependency.

Employment programs and educational resources further support recovery by providing purpose and focus beyond the immediate realm of addiction. By enabling individuals to engage in meaningful work and personal development activities, these services foster a sense of achievement and self-worth that can fortify sobriety.

Let us not forget the power of personal responsibility and self-care in this equation. Taking ownership of one's health and recovery can be transformative. It involves setting goals, reflecting on progress, and celebrating victories, no matter how small. Remember, a series of small steps can amount to a monumental journey.

Lastly, it is important to recognize that setbacks may occur. Relapse should not be viewed as a failure but as an opportunity for learning and growth. The recovery path is unique for everyone, and perseverance coupled with the right support can lead to a lifetime of better health and freedom from addiction—true victories for heart health.

Rising above substance abuse is a testament to the human spirit's resilience. It embodies a fundamental aspect of heart health—recognizing the power we hold to change our trajectory and then taking the steps, though they may be arduous, toward wellness and vitality. Recovery is possible, and a heart-healthy life, free from the shackles of substance abuse, awaits.

Chapter 12:
Mental Health and Its Impact on Heart Health

As we delve deeper into the essence of whole-body wellness, we recognize the profound intertwine of mental health with the vitality of our hearts. It's long been established how stress, anxiety, and depression tread not so silently on the periphery of cardiovascular disease. In this chapter, we navigate through the evidence-backed links that bind our emotional well-being to the core of heart health. We'll uncover strategies for managing stress, nuanced techniques designed to mitigate its erosive effects on our cardiac function. Moreover, this exploration is an invitation to honor and process our psychological landscape as an essential aspect of heart disease prevention and management. Mental resilience isn't just about strength—it's about recognizing vulnerability as the first step towards transformation, offering a lifeline to not only mend broken spirits but also to fortify the beating heart against the tempests of life.

The Connection Between Mental Health and Heart Disease

The intricate interplay between mental health and heart disease is a realm where emotions and the cardiovascular system converge. This section highlights the considerable evidence suggesting that mental health significantly influences heart health. It's crucial to understand that the heart isn't just an organ pumping blood; it can also be profoundly impacted by our emotional and psychological well-being.

Mental health disorders such as depression and anxiety are not just confined to the mind as we once thought. They bear a tangible impact on the body, particularly the heart. Individuals with depression have been found to possess an elevated risk of developing heart disease. This isn't purely a correlation; it includes direct and indirect physiological effects that depression imposes onto heart function and structure. Depression can alter the nervous system responses, leading to increased heart rate and blood pressure, markers that are linked to heart disease.

Anxiety, too, shares a notorious link with heart disease. The heightened state of alert and physiological arousal that comes with anxiety disorders can place an excessive strain on the heart. The persistent elevation of stress hormones, such as cortisol and adrenaline, can wreak havoc on the cardiovascular system, increasing the risk of hypertension and subsequent heart disease down the line.

Stress, a pervasive aspect of modern life, is another mental health concern that is tightly woven with heart health. Chronic stress can lead to behaviors that exacerbate heart disease risk, such as poor dietary habits, smoking, and neglecting exercise. Moreover, chronic stress itself can trigger inflammatory responses that are harmful to blood vessels and may contribute to plaque buildup, known as atherosclerosis.

Elucidating the link between mental health and heart disease also requires us to delve into the complexities of psychosocial factors. Factors like social isolation, loneliness, and lack of social support can negatively impact heart health. These conditions do not merely affect emotional well-being but can have measurable effects on heart rate variability and other cardiac risk markers.

The phenomenon of "broken heart syndrome," also known as Takotsubo cardiomyopathy, embodies the extreme effect that acute emotional distress can have on the heart, sometimes mimicking a heart attack. This condition dramatically illustrates how sudden, intense emotional stress can lead to severe, but often reversible, heart muscle weakness.

Conversely, a robust mental state and the presence of positive emotions can have protective effects on the heart. Positivity, optimism, and a sense of purpose are associated with lower rates of heart disease. These elements seem to mitigate cardiovascular risk, partly through healthier lifestyles and possibly through direct physiological benefits.

It's also vital to consider the bidirectional nature of this relationship. Just as mental health issues can lead to heart disease, the experience of heart disease can greatly impact an individual's mental health. A heart disease diagnosis can be a significant psychological burden, leading to depression and anxiety, which can further complicate heart disease management.

Understanding these connections affords us the opportunity to use mental health interventions as a tool for heart disease prevention and management. Therapeutic approaches like cognitive-behavioral therapy (CBT), mindfulness-based therapies, and stress management techniques can substantially alleviate the burden on the heart by improving mental health.

Medications that are commonly prescribed for mental health conditions can have implications for heart disease as well. Certain antidepressants, for example, can influence heart rate and blood pressure, hence their use requires careful monitoring in individuals with or at risk of heart disease.

Self-care practices—including adequate sleep, stress reduction techniques, and fostering strong social connections—serve as important strategies for managing both mental and heart health. Good sleep hygiene is especially important, as poor sleep can be both a symptom of mental health issues and a contributor to heart disease.

Exercise emerges as a powerful tool that straddles the divide between mental and heart health. By promoting the release of endorphins, known as the body's natural mood lifters, and improving cardiovascular fitness, regular physical activity is indispensable in the fight against heart disease and the improvement of mental well-being.

The role of nutrition should not be overlooked either. A heart-healthy diet is inherently also beneficial for mental health, providing the brain and the heart with the nutrients needed for optimum performance. Omega-3 fatty acids, for instance, are just as crucial for cognitive function as they are for heart function.

In conclusion, addressing mental health is a critical, yet sometimes overlooked, component of heart disease prevention and management. It's essential to treat the mind and heart not as separate entities but as interconnected systems that both require care and attention. Through lifestyle modifications, therapeutic interventions, and social support, we can empower individuals to nurture their mental well-being alongside their heart health.

As we continue this exploration into mental health and heart disease, we'll delve into specific, actionable stress management techniques, underscoring their pivotal role in protecting the heart. After all, a balanced mind is a precursor to a healthy heart, charting a path toward a life of fulfillment and vitality.

Stress Management Techniques

Severing the ties between stress and heart disease is a battle fought with more than just medication; it's a campaign that demands lifestyle transformations and commitment. Integrating stress management techniques into one's daily routine can buffer the stealthy encroachments of stress on the heart. Mindfulness meditation, deep-breathing exercises, and progressive muscle relaxation stand as sentinels, safeguarding the heart by resetting the stress response. Visualization and guided imagery serve as empowering allies, helping to reconstruct a fortress of calm within the turbulent seas of day-to-day stressors. Time spent in nature, the adoption of yoga, or participation in Tai Chi are not mere pastimes; they are gatekeepers of tranquility, protecting against the onslaught of chronic stress known to fray the intricate networks of one's cardiovascular well-being. In cultivating these habits of tranquility, you're not merely escaping stress; you're constructing a sanctuary of heart health that resists the wear and tear of modern pressures.

Coping with Heart Disease: Psychological Aspects

Heart disease can be a life-altering diagnosis. It carries significant weight, not only on your physical well-being but also on your psychological state. As you strive for a healthier heart and lifestyle, acknowledging and addressing the emotional toll of heart disease is crucial. Grappling with heart disease requires resilience; understanding how to fortify your mental health is a significant step toward recovery and management.

Firstly, it is common to experience a range of emotions after being diagnosed with heart disease. These may include shock, denial, anger, depression, and anxiety. Such reactions are not only normal but are also manageable. Accepting these feelings as part of your journey towards a healthy heart is the initial step toward psychological well-being.

Open communication with your healthcare provider is invaluable. It facilitates a thorough understanding of your condition and eases anxiety. Knowledge is empowering. With clarity about your heart disease, you are better positioned to tackle it head-on and maintain a proactive stance toward your health.

Establishing a strong support system is equally vital. Lean on family, friends, or support groups who understand your challenges. These networks provide comfort and advice and can be instrumental in reducing feelings of isolation or sadness that may arise from dealing with chronic illness.

Stress management techniques, such as meditation, deep breathing exercises, and mindfulness, can significantly impact your psychological health. Integrating such practices into your daily routine can help alleviate stress and improve your overall sense of well-being. Remember that a relaxed mind can lead to a healthier heart.

Incorporating positive lifestyle changes, such as a balanced diet and regular exercise, not only benefits your heart condition but also improves your mood and energy levels. Exercise, in particular, releases endorphins, which are natural mood lifters. Plus, the sense of accomplishment from achieving fitness goals can bolster your mental health.

Cognitive behavioral therapy (CBT) is another effective method for coping with the emotional and mental challenges of heart disease. CBT can help alter negative thought patterns and develop more adaptive ways of thinking, empowering you to better handle the emotional toll of the condition.

Set realistic and achievable goals for yourself. Whether they focus on dietary changes, exercise regimens, or managing stress, these goals give you a sense of purpose and progression. Celebrate the small victories—they are proof of your commitment to well-being.

Remember that it's okay to seek professional help if you're struggling to cope. Mental health professionals specialize in helping individuals navigate the emotional responses associated with chronic illnesses, including heart disease. They can offer strategies tailored to your specific needs and circumstances.

Journaling or other forms of self-expression can be therapeutic outlets for emotions. Documenting your thoughts, fears, and triumphs provides a means to reflect on your experiences and can be cathartic, helping to ease inner turmoil.

Mindfulness and acceptance are key ingredients in the fight against heart disease. Cultivating a practice of living in the present moment reduces worries about the future and regrets from the past. Accepting the present as it is, without judgment, can lessen fear and anxiety.

Education is empowerment. Understanding your condition and the psychological effects associated with it will help you rationalize what you feel. Participate in educational workshops, attend seminars, or read up on the latest research. Accessing resources can provide both comfort and command over your situation.

Lastly, never underestimate the power of humor and positivity. They are not frivolous; they are vital tools for psychological well-being. Laughter can improve your immune system and relieve stress. A positive outlook can inspire hope, which is essential in the journey to heart health.

In closing, dealing with heart disease goes beyond physical treatments; it involves nurturing your psychological health. Taking charge of your emotional well-being is a critical element in combating heart disease and working towards a heart-healthy lifestyle, underscoring the interconnectedness of mind and body. Embrace each day with determination, and remember that every small step you take is progress on your path to a healthier heart—and a fulfilling life.

Chapter 13:
Empowering Your Heart-Healthy Journey

As we conclude this essential journey through the intricacies of heart health, it's important to remember that the power to effect change lies within each of us. You have explored the physical mechanics of your heart, understood the risks specific to men, and learned to recognize the critical signs that demand immediate attention. Armed with this knowledge, you're now positioned at the helm, ready to steer your life towards a heart-healthy future.

Transitioning from learning to doing isn't always an easy path, but it's undoubtedly a rewarding one. Lifestyle choices form the cornerstone of cardiac well-being. By choosing to quit smoking, managing stress effectively, and ensuring a restorative night's sleep, you're building a solid foundation for your heart to thrive upon.

Nutrition, too, is a mighty ally in this fight against heart disease. Embracing a heart-healthy diet isn't about a quick fix; it's about creating sustainable habits that become second nature. By incorporating nutrient-dense foods and being mindful of those to avoid, along with understanding the role of supplements, you're fueling your body with what it truly needs to combat heart disease.

Let's not forget the vitality of regular exercise. A stronger heart is one that beats with vigor, supported by the benefits of physical activity. The creation of a personalized exercise plan is not about rigorous demands; it's about weaving activity into your daily life in ways that you enjoy, ensuring that motivation remains high for the long-term journey.

Managing weight is another battlefront in the war against heart disease. By understanding the link between weight and heart health, and adopting strategies for losing weight safely, you empower yourself to make informed decisions that have a profound impact on your wellbeing.

The importance of managing blood pressure and cholesterol can't be overstated. Through vigilant monitoring and adopting strategies to keep these in check, you'll greatly reduce your risk factors. Consistent health screenings serve as a compass, guiding you towards the path of lasting heart health.

Even as diabetes presents a formidable challenge, it is one that is surmountable. By focusing on lifestyle management, monitoring, and medication compliance, the link between diabetes and heart disease can be weakened, providing you with a fighting chance for a healthier heart.

Facing the dangers of alcohol and drugs requires courage and earnest self-reflection. Recognizing their effects on your heart and seeking help for substance abuse, if needed, is a courageous step towards safeguarding your heart's health.

The interconnectedness of mental health and heart disease underscores the importance of adopting effective stress management techniques. Learning to cope well with heart disease from a psychological standpoint isn't just beneficial; it's a critical aspect of your overall heart care plan.

The onward march doesn't end here; it's a continuous voyage that will have its storms and its calms. As with any journey, there will be moments of doubt, but also times of exhilarating triumph. Remember that every step you take towards a healthier heart is a step in the right direction, no matter how small it may seem.

Your heart-healthy journey is deeply personal and uniquely yours, but it's also a shared experience with millions of others, each with their own stories, challenges, and victories. Community and support are invaluable resources—never hesitate to reach out to support groups, healthcare professionals, friends, and family who can offer guidance, encouragement, and companionship.

You've armed yourself with knowledge and strategies rich in potential. They are the compass and map you need to navigate through the complexities of heart disease. The decisions you make from this point forward have power—the power to shape not just the quantity of your years, but the quality of your life.

May this book serve as a beacon of hope and a reminder that while the journey is yours, you're far from alone. Remember to revisit the elements of this guide as often as necessary. As life evolves, so too may your approach to maintaining heart health. The pages herein are designed to grow with you, offering timeless insights and advice that remain relevant at every stage of your life.

With every heartbeat, let yourself be inspired by the remarkable capacity for renewal and resilience that lies within. Your heart is an incredible powerhouse, and with care, attention, and dedication, it can propel you towards a future rich with vitality and joy.

In closing, grasp the reins of this empowering journey with both hands. With each heart-healthy choice, envision the vibrant life you're fostering—an existence not defined by heart disease, but by the strength and courage to rise above it. May this book not be the end, but rather a vibrant new beginning to a heart-healthy life full of potential, passion, and purpose.

Appendix A:
Heart-Healthy Recipes

Embarking on a journey toward heart health doesn't mean sacrificing the joy of delicious meals. It's about discovering new flavors, textures, and culinary experiences that not only satisfy your palate but also nurture your heart. The recipes provided in this Appendix are crafted with care to ensure they are as nutritious as they are flavorful, demonstrating that heart-healthy eating can be a delightful and sustainable part of your lifestyle.

Hearty Oatmeal with Berries and Nuts

- **Ingredients:** 1 cup rolled oats, 2 cups water or almond milk, 1/2 cup mixed berries, 1/4 cup chopped walnuts, 1 tablespoon ground flaxseed, a drizzle of honey or pure maple syrup (optional)

- **Instructions:** In a medium saucepan, bring water or almond milk to a boil. Add oats and reduce heat. Let simmer, stirring occasionally, until the oats are soft and have absorbed most of the liquid. Remove from heat and stir in berries, walnuts, and flaxseed. Sweeten with honey or maple syrup if desired. Serve warm.

Grilled Salmon with Steamed Broccoli

- **Ingredients:** 2 salmon fillets (4 oz each), 1 tablespoon olive oil, 1 teaspoon lemon zest, 1 tablespoon lemon juice, 2 cups broccoli florets, salt, and pepper to taste

- **Instructions:** Preheat the grill to medium-high heat. Brush salmon with olive oil and sprinkle with lemon zest, lemon juice, salt, and pepper. Grill the salmon for 4-5 minutes on each side or until cooked through. Meanwhile, steam broccoli until tender yet still crisp. Serve salmon with a side of steamed broccoli.

Quinoa and Black Bean Salad

- **Ingredients:** 1 cup quinoa, 2 cups water, 1 can black beans (drained and rinsed), 1 large tomato (chopped), 1 avocado (chopped), 1/4 cup red onion (finely chopped), 1/4 cup cilantro (chopped), 2 tablespoons olive oil, juice of 1 lime, salt, and pepper to taste

- **Instructions:** Rinse quinoa in a fine-mesh strainer. In a saucepan, bring water to boil. Add quinoa and reduce heat to low. Cover and simmer for 15-20 minutes or until quinoa is tender and water is absorbed. Let cool. In a large bowl, combine cooled quinoa, black beans, tomato, avocado, red onion, and cilantro. Drizzle with olive oil and lime juice, toss to combine, and season with salt and pepper.

Vegetable Stir-Fry Over Brown Rice

- **Ingredients:** 1 cup brown rice, 2 tablespoons olive oil, 2 cups assortment of bell peppers, broccoli, snap peas, and carrots (sliced), 2 cloves garlic (minced), 2 tablespoons low-sodium soy sauce or tamari, 1 tablespoon sesame oil, sesame seeds (for garnish)

- **Instructions:** Cook brown rice according to package instructions. Heat olive oil in a wok or large skillet over medium-high heat. Add vegetables and garlic, stirring frequently, and cook until they're vibrant and slightly tender. Add soy sauce or tamari and cook for an additional minute. Drizzle with sesame oil. Serve the stir-fry over the cooked brown rice and sprinkle with sesame seeds.

To close, embracing heart-healthy eating habits isn't about limiting your culinary world; it's about expanding it with mindful choices. These recipes are designed to fuel your body and bring joy to your table. They're a wonderful blend of wholesome ingredients, proving that food that's good for your heart can also be incredibly satisfying. So, treat your heart well with these scrumptious, nutrient-packed meals, and remember that every bite is a step towards a healthier you.

Appendix B:
Recommended Exercise Routines

Embarking on a journey toward better heart health, exercise is a cornerstone not only for its physical benefits but also for the mental and emotional resilience it fosters. In the following guide, you'll find exercise routines designed to cater to various levels of fitness and cardiac health. Keep in mind, it's essential to seek advice from your healthcare provider before starting any new exercise regimen, especially if you're managing heart disease or any other medical conditions.

Getting Started

The key to sustainable exercise is steady progression. Begin with lighter activities and gradually increase intensity as your fitness improves. Initially, focus on frequency rather than duration or intensity to establish a consistent exercise habit. Walking is a fantastic starting point—aim for a brisk pace, but ensure you can maintain a conversation without gasping for breath.

Low-Intensity Exercises

- **Walking:** Aim for at least 30 minutes a day, five times a week. Walking is highly adaptable; it can be done indoors on a treadmill or outdoors in a park or around your neighborhood.

- **Swimming:** Gentle on the joints and beneficial for endurance, swimming for 30 minutes at a comfortable pace is a great low-impact workout.

- **Cycling:** A stationary bike can provide an excellent cardio-vascular workout. Start with 15–20 minutes and increase the duration as your endurance builds.

Moderate-Intensity Exercises

As your body adapts, incorporate moderate-intensity exercises into your routine. These should be challenging yet doable, elevating your heart rate and breathing while still allowing you to hold a conversation.

- **Brisk Walking or Jogging:** Transition from a walk to a light jog, aiming for a pace that gets your heart pumping but isn't overly strenuous.

- **Aerobics:** Low-impact aerobics classes can help build stamina and muscle strength. Find a class that caters to heart patients or those looking for a gentler approach.

- **Dance:** Join a dance class or just dance at home to your favorite tunes for around 30 minutes to get a fun and effective workout.

Strength Training

Twice a week, introduce strength training to build muscle, support joints, and improve overall heart function. Use light weights or resistance bands, focusing on major muscle groups. Perform two sets of 10–12 repetitions for each exercise, ensuring that you don't hold your breath as you exert effort; exhale on the work phase and inhale on the release.

Flexibility and Balance

Incorporate stretching or yoga at least once or twice a week to improve flexibility and balance, which are crucial for overall functional fitness and can help prevent falls.

Examples of Strength Training Exercises

- **Wall Push-ups:** Stand an arm's length from a wall, place your hands on the wall at shoulder height and width, then perform push-ups against the wall.

- **Chair Squats:** Stand in front of a chair with feet shoulder-width apart, lower your body back as if to sit, touch the chair's edge lightly, and stand back up.

- **Bicep Curls:** With a light dumbbell in each hand, curl the weights toward your shoulders while keeping your elbows close to your body.

Consistency is Key

It's not about having one intense workout; rather, it's about consistent, moderate activity. Strive for a balance of cardiovascular, strength, flexibility, and balance exercises throughout the week for a holistic approach. Track your progress and celebrate the victories, no matter how small. Remember, every step taken is a step closer to a healthier heart and a more vibrant life.

As you adopt these exercise routines, listen keenly to your body's signals, appreciating your capabilities and respecting your limits. Through patient and persistent effort, you can significantly enhance your heart's health and vitality. Let these exercises be a testimony to the strength within you, proving that a heart condition doesn't define your potential; it merely sets the stage for a triumphant rise.

Appendix C:
Resources for Heart Health and Support Groups

Empowering your journey towards a heart-healthy lifestyle is not just about individual initiative; it's also about the strength you can draw from the support and information available around you. This section provides a curated list of resources that can be a lifeline for men living with heart disease, their caregivers, and anyone else committed to heart health.

National and International Organizations

1. American Heart Association (AHA)

- Offers valuable information on heart disease, including educational resources, dietary recommendations, and an extensive network of local support groups.

2. World Heart Federation

- Connects patients, doctors, and policymakers globally to fight against cardiovascular disease.

3. National Heart, Lung, and Blood Institute (NHLBI)

- Provides guidelines and research on heart health, and is a hub for clinical trials and the latest in heart health science.

Support Networks and Groups

1. Mended Hearts

- An organization offering peer-to-peer support for heart disease patients, caregivers, and families.

2. WomenHeart: The National Coalition for Women with Heart Disease

- While focusing on women, this resource offers excellent comprehensive support that men can use, too, especially their educational materials and community programs.

3. Heart-Healthy Living Online Community

- A place to share your journey, ask questions, and seek motivation from others dedicated to living a heart-healthy life.

Online Resources and Tools

1. My Life Check by American Heart Association

- This tool helps to assess your heart health and create a personalized plan to improve it.

2. CDC Heart Disease

- The Centers for Disease Control and Prevention offer comprehensive statistics, fact sheets, and prevention strategies.

Apps and Tech for Heart Health

Incorporating heart health tracking into your daily routine can help keep you accountable and informed. There is a plethora of apps designed to track your dietary intake, physical activity, blood pressure, and even stress levels. While specifics won't be listed here, searching in app stores for "heart health" can provide you with numerous options to explore.

Educational Books and Materials

From understanding the complexities of heart disease to learning about diet and exercise, a range of books can provide insight and guidance. Look for titles that are backed by substantial research and authored by noted cardiologists or health experts. Your local library or bookstore can be an excellent starting point for discovering these materials.

Counseling and Therapy

Exploring the psychological impact of living with heart disease is just as crucial as the physical aspect. Seeking professional help through therapy can help you develop coping skills to manage stress, depression, or anxiety related to your condition.

In Conclusion

You are not alone on your quest for a healthier heart. Whether it's talking to others who've walked in your shoes, delving into the latest science about heart health, or simply finding your tribe in a local or online community, use these resources to their fullest potential. Your heart, your health, and your happiness are worth every effort you make, every piece of knowledge you gain, and every support you seek. Remember, maintaining heart health is a continuous journey — and these resources are your companions along the way.

www.ingramcontent.com/pod-product-compliance
Lightning Source LLC
Chambersburg PA
CBHW051447280526
45785CB00003B/1457